Social Work Practice with War-Affected Children

This book explores the effects of war and migration on individual children and their family system, and how culturally responsive social work practice should take into account the diversity and heterogeneity of their needs and lived experiences.

Unpacking social work practice with children and families affected by war and migration, the volume provides a valuable toolkit for practitioners, educators, researchers, and service-providers that work with war-affected populations around the globe. The contributions suggest that fostering a family approach, allotting careful attention to context and culture, and linking the arts and participation with social work practice can all be vital to enhancing the research, education, and practice around working with children and families affected by war and migration.

Providing a critical reflection of social work education and practice, this book will be of interest to practitioners in the field of social work, as well as researchers studying the social effects of migration.

This book was originally published as a special issue of the *Journal of Family Social Work*.

Myriam Denov is a Full Professor of Social Work at McGill University, Canada, and holds the Canada Research Chair in Youth, Gender and Armed Conflict. Her research centers on children and families affected by war, migration, and their intergenerational effects. She is the author of *Child Soldiers: Sierra Leone's Revolutionary United Front* (2010), and co-editor of *Children Affected by Armed Conflict: Theory, Method and Practice* (2017).

Meaghan C. Shevell holds a Bachelor of Arts in Anthropology and Psychology from McGill University, Canada, and a Master of Arts in Human Rights Studies from Columbia University, USA, where she specialized in children's rights in conflict settings.

Social Work Practice with War-Affected Children

The Importance of Family, Art, Culture, and Context

Edited by

Myriam Denov and Meaghan C. Shevell

Routledge
Taylor & Francis Group
LONDON AND NEW YORK

First published 2019
by Routledge
2 Park Square, Milton Park, Abingdon, Oxon, OX14 4RN

and by Routledge
52 Vanderbilt Avenue, New York, NY 10017

Routledge is an imprint of the Taylor & Francis Group, an informa business

British Library Cataloguing-in-Publication Data
A catalogue record for this book is available from the British Library

ISBN13: 978-0-367-27262-3

Typeset in Minion Pro
by codeMantra

Publisher's Note
The publisher accepts responsibility for any inconsistencies that may have arisen during the conversion of this book from journal articles to book chapters, namely the inclusion of journal terminology.

Disclaimer
Every effort has been made to contact copyright holders for their permission to reprint material in this book. The publishers would be grateful to hear from any copyright holder who is not here acknowledged and will undertake to rectify any errors or omissions in future editions of this book.

Contents

Citation Information

The chapters in this book were originally published in the *Journal of Family Social Work*, volume 22, issue 1 (January 2019). When citing this material, please use the original page numbering for each article, as follows:

Introduction
Social work practice with war-affected children and families: the importance of family, culture, arts, and participatory approaches
Myriam Denov and Meaghan C. Shevell
Journal of Family Social Work, volume 22, issue 1 (January 2019) pp. 1–16

Chapter 1
Intergenerational resilience in families affected by war, displacement, and migration: "It runs in the family"
Myriam Denov, Maya Fennig, Marjorie Aude Rabiau, and Meaghan C. Shevell
Journal of Family Social Work, volume 22, issue 1 (January 2019) pp. 17–45

Chapter 2
Rethinking the meaning of "family" for war-affected young people: implications for social work education
Natasha Blanchet-Cohen, Myriam Denov, Alusine Bah, Leontine Uwababyeyi, and Jean Kagame
Journal of Family Social Work, volume 22, issue 1 (January 2019) pp. 46–62

Chapter 3
Beginning at the beginning in social work education: a case for incorporating arts-based approaches to working with war-affected children and their families
Claudia Mitchell, Warren Linds, Myriam Denov, Miranda D'Amico, and Brenda Cleary
Journal of Family Social Work, volume 22, issue 1 (January 2019) pp. 63–82

Chapter 4
Culture, migration, and identity formation in adolescent refugees: a family perspective
Marjorie Aude Rabiau
Journal of Family Social Work, volume 22, issue 1 (January 2019) pp. 83–100

Chapter 5

The essential role of the father: fostering a father-inclusive practice approach with immigrant and refugee families
Sharon Bond
Journal of Family Social Work, volume 22, issue 1 (January 2019) pp. 101–123

Notes on Contributors

Alusine Bah is a student studying in Social Work at McGill University, Montreal, Canada.

Natasha Blanchet-Cohen is an Associate Professor in the Department of Applied Human Sciences at Concordia University, Montreal, Canada.

Sharon Bond is an Associate Professor in the McGill School of Social Work at McGill University, Montreal, Canada.

Brenda Cleary is completing her master's degree at Ingram School of Nursing at McGill University, Montreal, Canada.

Miranda D'Amico is a Professor in the Department of Education at Concordia University, Montreal, Canada.

Myriam Denov is a Full Professor of Social Work at McGill University, Montreal, Canada, and holds the Canada Research Chair in Youth, Gender and Armed Conflict.

Maya Fennig is a PhD Student in the School of Social Work at McGill University, Montreal, Canada.

Jean Kagame is a Student studying Social Work at McGill University, Montreal, Canada.

Warren Linds is an Associate Professor in the Department of Applied Human Sciences at Concordia University, Montreal, Canada.

Claudia Mitchell is a James McGill Professor in the Department of Integrated Studies in Education at McGill University, Montreal, Canada.

Marjorie Aude Rabiau is an Assistant Professor in the School of Social Work at McGill University, Montreal, Canada.

Meaghan C. Shevell holds a Bachelor of Arts in Anthropology and Psychology from McGill University, Montreal, Canada, and a Master of Arts in Human Rights Studies from Columbia University, New York City, USA.

Léontine Uwababyeyi is a recent graduate of the School of Social Work at McGill University, Montreal, Canada.

INTRODUCTION

Social work practice with war-affected children and families: the importance of family, culture, arts, and participatory approaches

Myriam Denov and Meaghan C. Shevell

ABSTRACT

War and armed conflict not only gravely impact individual children, but the entire family system, with the impacts of war further compounded by the complexities of displacement, flight, migration, and resettlement to new contexts. These processes can cause destabilizing ruptures in the social fabric, networks, and services that support and protect children and families, ultimately hindering their potential protective capacities and potentially contributing to negative long-term intergenerational effects. The family plays a vital role in shaping children's mental health and well-being in conflict and post conflict settings, and thus the family needs to be accorded greater consideration in designing psychosocial support services for war-affected populations. With growing numbers of war-affected refugees resettling in Canada and the U.S., it is critical that psychosocial programs and interventions address their unique needs, as individuals, families, and communities. Moreover, there is a greater need for culturally responsive practice with war-affected refugee children and families that accounts for the diversity and heterogeneity of their needs and lived experiences. In this Special Issue entitled: "Children of War and their Families: Perspectives on Social Work Practice & Education", we suggest that factors such as fostering a family approach, allotting careful attention to context and culture, alongside an emphasis on linking the arts and participation with social work practice, can be key social work contributions to research, education, and practice with this important and often overlooked population.

War and armed conflict form lasting impacts on children's physical, social, and psychological functioning and development and can lead to destabilizing ruptures in the social fabric, networks, and services that support well-being (Betancourt & Khan, 2008; UNICEF, 2009). These breakdowns in curative and preventative processes particularly hinder the protective capacities of the family, contributing to persisting intergenerational effects (Denov, 2015;

This article was originally published with errors, which have now been corrected in the online version. Please see Correction (http://dx.doi.org/10.1080/10522158.2019.1560949)

Devakumar, Birch, Osrin, Sondorp, & Wells, 2014). Importantly, war itself is not the only challenge and devastation. Displacement as a result of war, and its related consequences, are significant. The United Nations High Commissioner for Refugees (UNHCR, 2017a) estimates that 65.6 million people are forcibly displaced worldwide due to persecution, conflict, or human rights violations, which represents a record high in recent decades. Although children make up 31% of the global population, 51% of all forcibly displaced people are children (UNHCR, 2017a; 2017b).

War and armed conflict are global phenomena yet are intimately linked to North American children and families. Although wars may occur beyond U.S. and Canadian borders, each year, thousands of children enter both countries, fleeing from war zones (Betancourt et al., 2015; Stewart, 2011; Zong & Batalova, 2015). The United States and Canada have historically been global leaders in refugee resettlement.[1] The United States has been a significant refugee resettlement country, accepting more than three million refugees since 1975 (UNHCR, 2018). An influx of children fleeing violence seeking asylum in the United States has been evidenced at alarming rates, compelling the establishment of an in-country refugee/parole processing program for minors in 2015 to ensure their protected status (Dettlaff & Fong, 2016). In September 2016, the United States admitted 84,995 refugees, with the highest numbers of admissions coming from the Democratic Republic of Congo (16,370), followed by Syria (12,587), and Myanmar (12,347) (Krogstad & Radford, 2017). However, these numbers have been diminishing as a result of transformations currently underway in U.S. refugee policy under the Trump administration, which have been characterized by a rhetoric of rejection, exclusion, and restriction (Haines, Howell, & Keles, 2017). This reduction is evidenced in UNHCR's (2018) *US Refugee Resettlement Facts* which reports a substantial decrease since the preceding year, with numbers down to 53,716 refugees resettled to the United States in the 2017 fiscal year. Several authors (Cox, 2017; Goodkind & Hess, 2017; Hurley, 2017; Thomson, 2017) note that the Trump administration's "travel ban" executive orders have exacerbated existing barriers in seeking refuge in the United States, resulting in excessive deportation and detention, and effectively derailing resettlement efforts. In an extreme measure to try and track illegal immigration in the U.S., the Trump administration recently enacted a policy that effectively separated more than 1,600 migrant children from their parents to be housed in "cage-like detention centers" (The Guardian, 2018). Here, families are forcibly separated for months, without any mechanism or infrastructure in place to locate or reconnect the family.

Canada receives between 25,000 and 35,000 refugees every year. This represents about 10% to 12% of the roughly 250,000 permanent residents that settle in Canada annually (Citizenship and Immigration Canada, 2009). In 2016, UNHCR lauded Canada's resettlement of 46,700 refugees, a record high in refugees admitted since the implementation of the 1976 Immigration Act (UNHCR, 2017b). This represents a 133% increase compared to the previous year. Additionally, nearly one half (47%) of refugees admitted to Canada in 2016 were children (Immigration, Refugees, Citizenship Canada [IRCC], 2017). Currently, the Government of Canada reports a total of 50,380 asylum claimants processed across the country in 2017. Based on recent figures reported by the IRCC, as of January 29, 2017, Canada has resettled a total of 40,081 Syrian refugees (IRCC, 2017). This is due in part to Canada's humanitarian transfer of Syrian refugees with UNHCR's support, as part of the Canadian government's explicit commitment to resettle refugees with a "renewed focus on reuniting families" (IRCC, 2017). The government has also emphasized the importance of combined efforts with civil society and service providers to support refugees' resettlement and integration (UNHCR, 2017b).

With growing numbers of asylum claimants and their families receiving permanent residency and becoming interwoven in the North American social fabric, it is critical that psychosocial programs and interventions address their needs, as individuals, families, and communities. Moreover, there is a greater need for culturally responsive practice with war-affected refugee children and families that accounts for the diversity and heterogeneity of their needs and experiences.

A significant body of literature has focused on war-affected populations, highlighting the unique experiences of children and youth (Kingsley, 2017; Machel, 1996, 2001; Macosko, 2000; UNICEF, 2009), as well as the obstacles and challenges war-affected refugees must endure as a result of forced migration (Wilson, Murtaza, & Shakya, 2010). The impacts of war are often compounded by added stressors experienced in the displacement, relocation, migration, and resettlement process—whether in the home country prior to departure, in transit, upon arrival, as well as during the extended resettlement process (Derluyn & Broekaert, 2008; Fazel, Reed, Panter-Brick, & Stein, 2012).

Refugee children and families are at substantially higher risk than the general population for a variety of specific psychiatric disorders related to their exposure to war, violence, torture, and forced migration (Kirmayer et al., 2011; Wilson et al., 2010). Moreover, children who are separated from their families pre- or postmigration are said to be at increased risk of psychological and social challenges (Bean, Derluyn, Eurelings-Bontekoe, Broekaert, & Spinhoven, 2007; Hodes, Jagdev, Chandra, & Cunniff, 2008). Forced migration experiences are often characterized by disruption, loss, and rebuilding key social networks and thus risk lacking sufficient social support (Liamputtong & Kurban, 2018; Oppedal & Idsoe, 2015; Reed, Fazel, Jones, Panter-Brick, & Stein, 2012). For refugee children, war-related mental health distress may occur alongside poverty, discrimination, isolation, and school difficulties (Denov & Bryan, 2014; Ellis et al., 2008). Importantly, research has consistently shown that the mental health impact of armed conflict is compounded or alleviated by contexts of migration and resettlement, with postmigration stressors found to be as powerful a predictor of distress as the exposure to war itself (Miller & Rasmussen, 2017). In this sense, the mental health of refugees is powerfully influenced by war-related violence and loss combined with the conditions they encounter en route to and within their host countries.

Although research on war-affected populations, particularly children, has traditionally focused on risks and vulnerabilities—oftentimes at the cost of pathologizing children—there has been a progressive shift toward efforts to better understand what promotes resilience despite profound forms of war and migration-related adversity (Betancourt & Khan, 2008; Fernando & Ferrari, 2013; Kostelny & Wessells, 2013; Werner, 2012). Within this burgeoning literature, children are accorded more agency in contributing to their own development and well-being, situating children's voices at the center of analysis and understanding. In this way, children are viewed as "reflexive subjects" who actively negotiate and make meaning of the social spaces and relations around them (Chaudhry, 2017). Approaches that focus on resilience can offer key insight on meaningful areas for strategic intervention by bolstering protective processes identified within the child's social ecology (Betancourt & Khan, 2008; Shakya et al., 2014; Williams & Drury, 2011). However, it is important to note that caution needs to be taken in the attention scholars and practitioners accord to resilience. As Denov and Akesson (2017) note, just as there may be a danger to overemphasizing traumatic experiences and vulnerability of war-affected children, researchers and practitioners may risk overemphasizing resilience in children, assuming that all will or have the capacity to bounce back. As such, recognizing the dynamic interplay of capacity and adversity, trauma, and resilience—within unique sociocultural contexts are thus essential.

It is also vital to recognize that war and migration do not simply affect individual children, but the entire family system. Families are often displaced from their homes and separated from one another, and the associated emotional stress may impair the ability of adults to provide care and nurturance to young children (Betancourt et al., 2015). Here, it is important to acknowledge the fluid nature of "the family," in determining family construction or who constitutes "family members," and the meanings attached. For example, consideration of "the family" is not exclusive to blood/kinship or marital relations. This is particularly relevant to the realities of war-affected populations where family composition and structure may shift profoundly as a result of war. Keeping in mind such broad and expansive meanings of *family*, war affects children and their families in numerous ways, including a disruption to various traditional family systems of support, challenging psychosocial well-being and capacities to heal and cope (Boothby, 2008). Family history and disruptions to the family unit are significant factors in consideration of young refugees' mental health outcomes (Fazel et al., 2012). The mental health of parents remains intimately connected to children and vice versa. Family support and cohesion are related to better mental health for young refugees (Kovacev & Shute, 2004; Rousseau, Drapeau, & Platt, 2004), as is parental mental health (Hjern, Angel, & Jeppson, 1998). Annan, Blattman, and Horton (2006) underscored the integral role of the family in the healing and well-being of war-affected youth, with those with high levels of family connectedness and support found to have better social functioning and lower levels of distress.

Mental health issues, affecting a family's ability to function, can persist long after the conflict has ended. Family stressors such as low socioeconomic background, precariousness of status, limited employment opportunities, and lack of official language ability have all been linked to higher rates of child mental health problems and long-term developmental problems (Fazel et al., 2012), as well as lower educational outcomes. Betancourt et al. (2015) argued that given the vital role that family plays in shaping children's mental health in postconflict settings, policy makers and service providers must understand and take into consideration not only the war exposure histories and mental health of children and adolescents, but also the mental health of their adult caregivers.

Approaches to social work practice with war-affected children and families

Given its broad approach and careful consideration of context, social work as a profession and discipline, has a great deal to offer to research and practice with war-affected populations—within war and conflict settings, as well as following forced migration and resettlement. And yet, aside from a few articles (Baum, 2007; Bilotta & Denov, 2017; Bragin, Taaka, Adolphs, Gray, & Eibs, 2015; Bragin et al., 2016; Fennig & Denov, 2018; Nelson, Price, & Zubrzycki, 2017; Ramon, Campbell, Lindsay, McCrystal, & Baidoun, 2006; Yan & Anucha, 2017), relatively little has been written on social work practice with war-affected populations, particularly refugees. We suggest that a family approach, as well as attention to context and culture, alongside an emphasis on linking the arts with social work practice, can be key social work contributions to research, education, and practice with this important population. We address each of these below.

A family approach

Youth are nested in meaningful social spheres that interact to either mobilize risk factors or bolster protective factors to reinforce resilience and community stabilization (Boothby, 2008; Boothby, Strang, & Wessells, 2006; Wessells, 2002). To best support war-affected children, it is critical to assess existing protective capacities and deficits in the systems that surround them to form a "protective shield" to reduce the full impact of socioecological shocks, such as those posed by war and war-induced migration (Boothby, 2008). In this way, protective elements can be specifically supported to promote protective environments that help to mitigate risks confronting war-affected refugee youth and their families.

A family approach can be particularly helpful in identifying the various risk and protective factors present in the multiple supportive layers, or social ecologies, that surround children and youth. Bronfenbrenner's (1986, 2009) classic socioecological model purports that children's development is shaped by dynamic reciprocal processes at multiple levels of the human social ecology, such as within the family, community, and society. Several authors have applied this model to the realities of refugees to gain a more holistic understanding of refugee well-being. Miller and Rasco (2004) highlight the significance of interactional relationships between environmental demands and available adaptive resources on shaping refugee healing and adaptation. McGregor, Melvin, and Newman (2016) described the importance of family as a supportive factor, for emotional and social support during the resettlement process. The presence of family members can transform adversity into a source of strength, by aiding in the rebuilding of a meaningful universe. This strength may help ensure the psycho-social, cultural, and economic survival of the family and the larger group. The family therefore can act as an anchor, for emotional security and identity, in exile (Rousseau, Mekki-Berrada, & Moreau, 2001).

As noted above, it is also important to (re)consider the notion of *family* itself. The enormous societal changes in our increasingly globalized world require that social workers contend with the transformations of what constitutes "family" in their practice and education. Indeed, conventional conceptualizations of the nuclear family no longer reflect current family realities (Woodford, 2006, p. 136). This is particularly important when considering war-affected populations who may have lost their entire family, may be separated from family, and may create new family structures in the postwar and postmigration contexts—ones that are not simply based on traditional bloodlines and kinship structures (Denov & Blanchet-Cohen, 2014).

The importance of culture and context

Traditional approaches to refugee psychosocial support have overwhelmingly been dominated by Western perspectives, which center on individualism and individualistic approaches to practice, intervention, and treatment (Bilotta & Denov, 2017). The individualistic, sometimes pathologizing, and biomedical emphasis of many intervention services in the Global North may be highly ineffective (Di Tomasso, 2010), as they may be experienced by clients as isolating, overemphasizing trauma and adversity, and overlooking important cultural meanings and idioms of trauma, distress, and recovery (Blanchet-Cohen, Denov, Fraser, & Bilotta, 2017). Privileging individual, trauma-focused Western interventions may risk imposing ethnocentric assumptions and marginalizing indigenous conceptualizations, which can result in harmful power asymmetries between the "helpers" and the "helped" (Kostelny, 2006). Rather, it is critical that a "therapeutic alliance" through collaboration be established to discern clients' contextualized understanding of wellness, illness, and coping.

Western paradigms of intervention may neglect to unpack key concepts such as "childhood," "family," and "well-being" to reveal the ways in which they are socially constructed and culturally relative in their meaning and implications. *Culture* describes a shared social system of knowledge, beliefs, values, and assumptions continuously guiding and shaping our behavior and our interrelations (Baldwin et al., 2006; Geertz, 1973; Keesing, 1974; Kroeber & Kluckhohn, 1952). Culture gives meaning to the physical experience, acting as a prism through which we not only perceive, but also make sense of the world around us. As such, culture plays a prominent role in how individuals conceptualize and experience illness, healing, and coping. In their review of the mental health and psychosocial well-being of war-affected Syrians, Hassan et al. (2015) demonstrated that services aimed to mitigate experiences of illness and promote psychosocial well-being must be tailored to the particular culture and context of clientele to have effective and sustainable impacts. In their work with war-affected Syrians, careful consideration was given to individual expressions and idioms (e.g., of distress, of "the self," of well-being/health) specific to the Syrian context; for example, this included more generally the interconnectedness of somatic (body) and psychological (soul) symptoms, the use of specific metaphors to explain and express suffering, and a "sociocentric" and "cosmocentric" conceptualization of the self. Although specific to Syrian cultural frameworks, much can be learned from their consideration of local idioms of distress to recognize the many ways people experience "illness." Granting specific considerations to cultural systems of knowledge and contextualized explanatory models of illness is essential in social work, as they have critical implications for help-seeking behavior, treatment expectations and concerns, and coping.

Although many scholars have highlighted the dangers of privileging individual, trauma-focused approaches, particularly with war-affected populations (Miller, Kulkarni, & Kushner, 2006; Miller & Rasco, 2004), social work practice and education continue to over-rely on approaches premised on these same assumptions (Fennig & Denov, 2018; Houston, 2014). These examples highlight the ways in which clinical assessments must be grounded in cultural and social contexts; they must include an effort to interpret what clients' expressions of distress and coping mean within their particular context. Understanding these idioms and explanatory models of "(un)wellness" can better tailor design interventions to galvanize the individual and collective resilience, strengths, capacities, and resources identified. It is imperative that social work practitioners and educators actively reflect on their own professional explanatory models and cultural idioms (e.g., Western biomedical model) and how this might differ from their clients or students.

Art and social work practice

Social work as a profession has historically engaged with art. As far back as the settlement house movement in the late 1800s, social work has incorporated the arts in community action by forming partnerships with artists in addressing social issues and human challenges (Moxley & Feen, 2016). Yet the 20th century saw a powerful movement away from artistic endeavors, toward scientific methods, and standardized efficacy (Konrad, 2017). This approach has prevailed in contemporary social work where a focus on managerialism and mechanistic practices have resulted in what many see as the repression of social work as a creative endeavor (Huss & Sela-Amit, 2018). Given the tragedy of war and genocide, words and narrative alone often cannot adequately capture the realities and complexity of conflict and migration-related experiences. As such, researchers and practitioners are increasingly turning to the arts to enable multiple forms of expression, as well as for the therapeutic, restorative, and empowering qualities of arts-based techniques (D'Amico, Denov, Khan, Linds, & Akesson, 2016; Green & Denov, in press; Leavy, 2009). Although the merging of art, war, migration, and direct social work practice are growing and essential for clients and practitioners, greater understanding of how art can be used within the context of social work practice and education is vital.

"Productive unknowing": social work research and practice merging war, family, culture, art, and participation

Contributors to this special issue are part of a team of Montreal-based researchers,[2] working in a variety of national and global contexts (Canada, Cambodia, Colombia, Ethiopia, Sierra Leone, South Africa, Syria, the Democratic Republic of the Congo (DRC), northern Uganda, Rwanda) with war-affected children and using a family systems approach to practice, participatory research approaches, and arts-based methods, who came together as part of a Research Group on Children in Global Adversity to consider critical issues related to family, art, and participation in this work. In our discussions over the last 6 years, we began to raise what might be described as "productive unknowing" questions (Vasudevan, 2011) in relation to the realities of social work research and practice as it relates to war-affected populations. What is the state of the art with regard to social work research and practice with war-affected populations, particularly as they relate to children and families? How can social work as a profession better contribute to the overall well-being of children and families affected by war? Although we found a rich body of work on social work with children and families, we became interested in deepening an understanding of the research and practice with war-affected children and families, particularly as they relate to key themes of interest to our research group: art, participation, culture, family systems, and the education of future social workers and practitioners.

Although the research team comprises three distinct axes that each focus on a key area or approach for war-affected youth (i.e., arts-based approaches, socio-ecological frameworks, and participatory methods), the research group aims to integrate these often distinct bodies of knowledge through a synergistic effort. The compilation of this special issue is a product of such synergy; team members met regularly to discuss individual axes' unique contribution to the field as well as to forge important linkages between axes. Our goal has been to bring together a collection of articles that merge a number of different areas of expertise and approaches that engage in critical thought on social work research, education, and practice. Through an iterative and collaborative review process that involved continuous discussion and reflection with an interdisciplinary team, this special issue aims to consider and reflect on current social work praxis, and how it can expand, evolve, and innovate to better meet the needs of war-affected children and families.

This special issue explores social work's role, positionality and potential—in research, practice, and education—with regard to war-affected children and their families. Specifically, this collection of articles explores the three main themes addressed above. First, several articles unpack the notion of *family* when working with war-affected populations, highlighting traditional social work "blindspots" when it comes to family practice, research, and education, as well as areas of promise. Second, articles in this collection implicitly and explicitly address the critical role of culture and context when practicing with war-affected children and families. Finally, the collection draws attention to the role of art in social work practice and education. We suggest that art may hold a vital and important place in education and clinical practice with war-affected children and families, as well as provide practitioners with powerful tools of intervention, and client empowerment and support.

In the first article, *"Intergenerational Resilience in Families Affected by War, Displacement and Migration: "It Runs in the Family,"* Myriam Denov and colleagues Maya Fennig, Marjorie Rabiau, and Meaghan C. Shevell explore and address the intergenerational realities of war and the ways in which armed conflict and war-induced migration affect the entire family, often over generations. This includes an examination of the intergenerational impacts of war-related trauma, as well as efforts to further conceptualize intergenerational resilience. The authors draw upon the unique case of a war-affected young person and trace his protracted journey to Canada to exemplify intergenerational resilience. Despite the multiple obstacles and experiences of trauma encountered across the migration process—including in the context of war, forced displacement, flight, migration, and resettlement—this participant powerfully demonstrates the capacity for individuals to draw on valuable adaptive capacities transferred onto them from family members in order to overcome profound adversity.

The second article, "'Rethinking the Meaning of "Family' for War-Affected Young People: Implications for Social Work Education," Natasha Blanchet-Cohen, Myriam Denov, Alusine Bah, Léontine Uwababyeyi, and Jean Kagame examine how the experiences and realities of young people affected by war appear to challenge the "typical" portrayal of "family" in social work education. Using aspects of duoethnography as a method of inquiry, where war-affected social work students directly reflected upon their own classroom experiences, the article illustrates the challenges that war-affected social work students face during the course of their social work training, particularly in the context of social work curriculum. The article highlights the need to rethink not only the meaning of *family* within social work curriculum, pedagogy, and course content, but also the negative implications of not challenging traditional meanings of family, particularly for the overall well-being of war-affected students, for the professional development of educators, and the innovation and social justice initiatives of social work profession as a whole.

In "Beginning at the Beginning in Social Work Education: A case for Incorporating Arts-based Approaches to Working with War-Affected Children and Their Families," Claudia Mitchell, Warren Linds, Myriam Denov, Miranda D'Amico, and Brenda Cleary unpack the ways that arts-based approaches can be incorporated into social work education particularly in the context of preparing new social work researchers and social workers to work with war-affected children and their families. Drawing together two bodies of literature, the literature on the arts in social work education, and literature on the arts and war affected children and their families, the article offers a set of five pedagogical practices that align well with arts-based methodologies. These include, reflexivity, situating one's self, observation, ethical practice and taking action. The article ultimately demonstrates the strengths and limitations of merging art, family, war, and social work education.

The fourth article, "Culture, Migration, and Identity Formation in Adolescence: A Family Perspective," utilizes a cultural lens at the family level to examine cultural identity and identity formation in adolescents in postmigratory contexts. In this article, Marjorie Rabiau explores the use of cultural idioms of distress and acculturation processes embedded in the family to assist in interpreting symptoms of distress. Particular attention is paid to the protective role of the family in mitigating stressors and threats to identity and self-concept posed during migration and resettlement. Additionally, Rabiau underscores the responsibilities of social workers in establishing safe therapeutic spaces and provides recommendations for capacity-strengthening efforts.

In the final article, "The Essential Role of the Father: Fostering a Father-Inclusive Approach with Immigrant and Refugee Families," Sharon Bond highlights the essential role of the father in immigrant and refugee children's psychosocial well-being, functioning, and development. Bond demonstrates how fathers have frequently been excluded from mainstream clinical social work practice, despite the critical role fathers play in child development. The lack of engagement with fathers is especially prominent among immigrant and refugee fathers, with psychosocial support services typically targeting women and their children. Bond highlights the various challenges and obstacles fathers face in accessing meaningful an supportive clinical services, while demonstrating the resilience of immigrant fathers and how father involvement can serve as a protective factor in the resilience and well-being of war-affected refugee youth and their families. Finally, Bond provides guidelines for father-inclusive practice, using a culturally-informed socioecological family systems model.

With the global plight of war-affected refugees on the rise, it is critical that social services offered in resettlement countries are relevant and pertinent to their unique needs. There is also a need for deeper reflection on one's own positionality as a practitioner, and how this shapes praxis. In addition, social work can benefit from a careful unpacking of key concepts that form the crux of practice and interventions, including health, well-being, illness, distress, healing, and family. The articles in this special issue highlight the importance of social work education according explicit attention to culture by embedding it into practice that can align well with arts-based approaches and contribute toward a more nuanced understanding of the multitude of ways individual and family experiences, conceptualizations, and meanings are shaped by the context in which we live. Ultimately, this contextualized knowledge can help improve the scope and reach of social work practice, curriculum development and pedagogy, by informing adaptations that ensure they are culturally relevant, appropriate and sensitive to the realities of war-affected children and their families.

Notes

1. The Canadian Council for Refugees asserts that Canada is one of the top three global leaders in refugee resettlement countries, with the private sponsorship of refugees a program unique to Canada.
2. Dr. Myriam Denov and a multidisciplinary team of Canadian researchers launched this multi-institutional research group in 2012. Funded by Fonds de recherche du Québec-Société et culture (FRQSC), this research group aims to explore the complex realities of war-affected children and families nationally and internationally.

Disclosure statement

No potential conflict of interest was reported by the authors.

References

Annan, J., Blattman, C., & Horton, R. (2006). *The state of youth and youth protection in Northern Uganda* (pp. 23). Uganda: UNICEF.

Baldwin, J. R., Faulkner, S. L., Hecht, M. L., & Lindsley, S. L. (Eds.). (2006). *Redefining culture: Perspectives across the disciplines*. London, UK: Routledge.

Baum, N. (2007). Social work practice in conflict-ridden areas: Cultural sensitivity is not enough. *British Journal of Social Work, 37*(5), 873–891. doi:10.1093/bjsw/bcl050

Bean, T., Derluyn, I., Eurelings-Bontekoe, E., Broekaert, E., & Spinhoven, P. (2007). Comparing psychological distress, traumatic stress reactions, and experiences of unaccompanied refugee minors with experiences of adolescents accompanied by parents. *The Journal of Nervous and Mental Disease, 195*(4), 288–297. doi:10.1097/01.nmd.0000243751.49499.93

Betancourt, T. S., Abdi, S., Ito, B. S., Lilienthal, G. M., Agalab, N., & Ellis, H. (2015). We left one war and came to another: Resource loss, acculturative stress, and caregiver–Child relationships in Somali refugee families. *Cultural Diversity and Ethnic Minority Psychology, 21*(1), 114. doi:10.1037/a0037538

Betancourt, T. S., & Khan, K. T. (2008). The mental health of children affected by armed conflict: Protective processes and pathways to resilience. *International Review of Psychiatry, 20*(3), 317–328. doi:10.1080/09540260802090363

Bilotta, N., & Denov, M. (2017). Theoretical understandings of unaccompanied young people affected by war: Bridging divides and embracing local ways of knowing. *The British Journal of Social Work, 48*(6).

Blanchet-Cohen, N., Denov, M., Fraser, S., & Bilotta, N. (2017). The nexus of war, resettlement, and education: War-affected youth's perspectives and responses to the Quebec education system. *International Journal of Intercultural Relations, 60*, 160–168. doi:10.1016/j.ijintrel.2017.04.016

Boothby, N. (2008). Political violence and development: An ecologic approach to children in war zones. *Child and Adolescent Psychiatric Clinics, 17*(3), 497–514. doi:10.1016/j.chc.2008.02.004

Boothby, N., Strang, A., & Wessells, M. (2006). *A world turned upside down: Social ecological approaches to children in war zones*. Bloomfield, CT: Kumarian Press.

Bragin, M., Taaka, J., Adolphs, K., Gray, H., & Eibs, T. (2015). Measuring difficult-to-measure concepts in clinical social work practice operationalizing psychosocial well-being among war-affected women: A case study in Northern Uganda. *Clinical Social Work Journal, 43*(4), 348–361. doi:10.1007/s10615-014-0507-0

Bragin, M., Tosone, C., Ihrig, E., Mollere, V., Niazi, A., & Mayel, E. (2016). Building culturally relevant social work for children in the midst of armed conflict: Applying the DACUM method in Afghanistan. *International Social Work, 59*(6), 745–759. doi:10.1177/0020872814527631

Bronfenbrenner, U. (1986). Ecology of the family as a context for human development: Research perspectives. *Developmental Psychology, 22*(6), 723. doi:10.1037/0012-1649.22.6.723

Bronfenbrenner, U. (2009). *The ecology of human development*. Cambridge, MA: Harvard University Press.

Chaudhry, L. (2017). "Raising the dead" and cultivating resilience: Postcolonial theory and children's narratives from Swat, Pakistan. In B. Akesson & M. Denov (Eds.), *Children affected by armed conflict: Theory, method, and practice* (pp. 23–42). New York Chichester, West Sussex: Columbia University Press.

Citizenship and Immigration Canada. (2009). Facts and figures: Immigration overview: Permanent and temporary residents 2008. Retrieved from http://www.cic.gc.ca/english/pdf/research-stats/facts2008.pdf

Cox, N. (2017). No safe place for someone like me: African Muslim asylum seekers react to Trump. In D. Haines, J. Howell, & F. Keles (Eds.), *Maintaining refuge: Anthropological reflections in uncertain times* (pp. 147–156). American Anthropological Association: A Publication of the Committee on Refugees and Immigrants.

D'Amico, M., Denov, M., Khan, F., Linds, W., & Akesson, B. (2016). Research as intervention? Exploring the health and well-being of children and youth facing global adversity through participatory visual methods. *Global Public Health*, *11*(5–6), 528–545. doi:10.1080/17441692.2016.1165719

Denov, M. (2015). Children born of wartime rape: The intergenerational realities of sexual violence and abuse. *Ethics, Medicine and Public Health*, *1*(1), 61–68. doi:10.1016/j.jemep.2015.02.001

Denov, M., & Akesson, B. (Eds.). (2017). *Children affected by armed conflict: Theory, method, and practice.* New York Chichester, West Sussex: Columbia University Press.

Denov, M., & Blanchet-Cohen, N. (2014). The rights and realities of war-affected refugee children and youth in Quebec: Making children's rights meaningful. Theme Issue, "Looking back, moving forward: Reflecting on 25 years of the convention on the rights of the child. *Canadian Journal for Children's Rights*, *1*(1), 18–43.

Denov, M., & Bryan, C. (2014). Social navigation and the resettlement experiences of separated children in Canada. *Refuge: Canada's Journal on Refugees*, *30*(1), 25–35.

Derluyn, I., & Broekaert, E. (2008). Unaccompanied refugee children and adolescent: The glaring contrast between a legal and a psychological perspective. *International Journal of Law and Psychiatry*, *31*(4), 319–330. doi:10.1016/j.ijlp.2007.11.006

Dettlaff, A., & Fong, R. (Eds.). (2016). *Immigrant and refugee children and families: Culturally responsive practice.* New York Chichester, West Sussex: Columbia University Press.

Devakumar, D., Birch, M., Osrin, D., Sondorp, E., & Wells, J. C. (2014). The intergenerational effects of war on the health of children. *BMC Medicine*, *12*, 57. doi:10.1186/s12916-014-0141-2

Di Tomasso, T. (2010). Approaches to counselling resettled refugee and asylum seeker survivors of organized violence. *International Journal of Child, Youth and Family Studies*, *1*(3/4), 244–264.

Ellis, B. H., MacDonald, H. Z., Lincoln, A. K., & Cabral, H. J. (2008). Mental health of Somali adolescent refugees: The role of trauma, stress, and perceived discrimination. *Journal of Consulting and Clinical Psychology*, *76*(2), 184. doi:10.1037/0022-006X.76.2.341

Fazel, M., Reed, R. V., Panter-Brick, C., & Stein, A. (2012). Mental health of displaced and refugee children resettled in high-income countries: Risk and protective factors. *Lancet*, *379*(9812), 266–282. doi:10.1016/S0140-6736(11)60051-2

Fennig, M., & Denov, M. (2018). Regime of Truth: Rethinking the Dominance of the bio-medical model in mental health social work with refugee youth. *British Journal of Social Work*, 1–18. doi:10.1093/bjsw/bcy036

Fernando, C., & Ferrari, M. (Eds.). (2013). *Handbook of resilience in children of war.* New York, NY: Springer Science & Business Media.

Geertz, C. (1973). *The interpretation of cultures* (Vol. 5019). New York, NY: Basic books.

Goodkind, J. R., & Hess, J. M. (2017). Refugee well-being project: A model for creating and maintaining communities of refuge in the United States. In D. Haines, J. Howell, & F. Keles (Eds.), *Maintaining refuge: Anthropological reflections in uncertain times* (pp. 139–146). New York Chichester, West Sussex: American Anthropological Association: A Publication of the Committee on Refugees and Immigrants.

Green, A., & Denov, M. (in press). Mask-making and drawing as method: An arts-based approach to data collection with war-affected children. *International Journal of Qualitative Research.*

Haines, D., Howell, J., & Keles, F. (2017). *Maintaining refuge: Anthropological reflections in uncertain times.* New York Chichester, West Sussex: American Anthropological Association: A Publication of the Committee on Refugees and Immigrants.

Hassan, G., Kirmayer, L. J., Mekki- Berrada, A., Quosh, C., El Chammay, R., Deville-Stoetzel, J. B., … Ventevogel, P. (2015). *Culture, context and the mental health and psychosocial wellbeing of Syrians: A review for mental health and psychosocial support staff working with Syrians affected by armed conflict.* Geneva, Switzerland: UNHCR.

Hjern, A., Angel, B., & Jeppson, O. (1998). Political violence, family stress and mental health of refugee children in exile. *Scandinavian Journal of Social Medicine, 26*(1), 18–25.

Hodes, M., Jagdev, D., Chandra, N., & Cunniff, A. (2008). Risk and resilience for psychological distress amongst unaccompanied asylum seeking adolescents. *Journal of Child Psychology and Psychiatry, 49*(7), 723–732. doi:10.1111/j.1469-7610.2008.01912.x

Holpuch, A. (2018, June 19). Families divided at the border: 'The most horrific immigration policy I've ever seen'. Retrieved from https://www.theguardian.com/us-news/2018/jun/19/families-border-separations-trump-immigration-policy

Houston, S. (2014). Beyond individualism: Social work and social identity. *The British Journal of Social Work, 46*(2), 532–548. doi:10.1093/bjsw/bcu097

Hurley, L. (2017). Trump travel ban fight heads towards Supreme Court showdown. *Reuters.* Retrieved May, 27 from http://www.reuters.com/article/us-usa-immigration-court-idUSKBN18M2C7

Huss, E., & Sela-Amit, M. (2018). Art in social work: Do we really need it? *Research on Social Work Practice,* doi: 10.1177/1049731517745995.

Immigration, Refugees, Citizenship Canada. (2017, November 1). *2017 Annual Report to Parliament on Immigration.* Retrieved from https://www.canada.ca/en/immigration-refugees-citizenship/corporate/publications-manuals/annual-report-parliament-immigration-2017.html#aboutThisReport

Keesing, R. M. (1974). Theories of culture. *Annual Review of Anthropology, 3*(1), 73–97. doi:10.1146/annurev.an.03.100174.000445

Kingsley, B. V. (2017). The effects that war has on children and child soldiers. *Senior Honors Theses.* 527. Retrieved from http://commons.emich.edu/honors/527

Kirmayer, L. J., Narasiah, L., Munoz, M., Rashid, M., Ryder, A. G., Guzder, J., … Pottie, K. (2011). Common mental health problems in immigrants and refugees: General approach in primary care. *Canadian Medical Association Journal, 183*(12), E959–E967. doi:10.1503/cmaj.090292

Konrad, S. C. (2017). Art in social work: Equivocation, evidence, and ethical quandaries. *Research on Social Work Practice.* doi:10.1177/1049731517735898

Kostelny, K. (2006). A culture-based, integrative approach. In N. Boothby, A. Strang, & M. Wessells (Eds.), *A world turned upside down: Social ecological approaches to children in war zones* (pp. 19–38). Bloomfield, CT: Kumarian Press.

Kostelny, K., & Wessells, M. (2013). Child friendly spaces: Promoting children's resiliency amidst war. In Fernando, C., & Ferrari, M. (Eds.), *Handbook of Resilience in Children of War* (pp. 119–129). New York, NY: Springer.

Kovacev, L., & Shute, R. (2004). Acculturation and social support in relation to psychosocial adjustment of adolescent refugees resettled in Australia. *International Journal of Behavioral Development, 28*(3), 259–267. doi:10.1080/01650250344000497

Kroeber, A., & Kluckhohn, C. (1952). Culture: A critical review of concepts and definitions (Papers of the peabody museum of american archaeology and ethnology, harvard university, v. 47, no. 1). Cambridge, Mass: Museum.

Krogstad, J. M., & Radford, J. (2017, January 30). *Key facts about refugees to the U.S.* Pew Research Center. Washington, DC. Retrieved from http://www.pewresearch.org/fact-tank/2017/01/30/key-facts-about-refugees-to-the-u-s/

Leavy, P. (2009). Arts-based research as a pedagogical tool for teaching media literacy: Reflections from an undergraduate classroom. *LEARNing Landscapes*, *3*(1), 225–242.

Liamputtong, P., & Kurban, H. (2018). Health, social integration and social support: The lived experiences of young Middle-Eastern refugees living in Melbourne, Australia. *Children and Youth Services Review*, *85*, 99–106. doi:10.1016/j.childyouth.2017.12.020

Machel, G. (1996). *Impact of armed conflict on children* (pp. 35). New York, NY: UN.

Machel, G. (2001). *The impact of war on children: A review of progress since the 1996 United Nations report on the impact of armed conflict on children.* United Nations Children's Fund, 3 UN Plaza, New York, NY 10017.

Macosko, E. (2000). Children of war: Conflict's impact on youth. *Harvard International Review*, *22*(3), 12–13. Retrieved from http://www.jstor.org/stable/42762626

McGregor, L. S., Melvin, G. A., & Newman, L. K. (2016). An exploration of the adaptation and development after persecution and trauma (ADAPT) model with resettled refugee adolescents in Australia: A qualitative study. *Transcultural Psychiatry*, *53*(3), 347–367. doi:10.1177/1363461516649546

Miller, K. E., Kulkarni, M., & Kushner, H. (2006). Beyond trauma-focused psychiatric epidemiology: Bridging research and practice with war-affected populations. *American Journal of Orthopsychiatry*, *76*(4), 409. doi:10.1037/0002-9432.76.4.409

Miller, K. E., & Rasco, L. M. (Eds.). (2004). *The mental health of refugees: Ecological approaches to healing and adaptation.* Mahwah, New Jersey: Taylor & Francis.

Miller, K. E., & Rasmussen, A. (2017). The mental health of civilians displaced by armed conflict: An ecological model of refugee distress. *Epidemiology and Psychiatric Sciences*, *26* (2), 129–138. doi:10.1017/S2045796016000172

Moxley, D. P., & Feen, H. (2016). Arts-inspired design in the development of helping interventions in social work: Implications for the integration of research and practice. *British Journal of Social Work*, *46*(6). doi:10.1093/bjsw/bcv087

Nelson, D., Price, E., & Zubrzycki, J. (2017). Critical social work with unaccompanied asylum-seeking young people: Restoring hope, agency and meaning for the client and worker. *International Social Work*, *60*(3), 601–613. doi:10.1177/0020872816637663

Oppedal, B., & Idsoe, T. (2015). The role of social support in the acculturation and mental health of unaccompanied minor asylum seekers. *Scandinavian Journal of Psychology*, *56*(2), 203–211. doi:10.1111/sjop.12194

Ramon, S., Campbell, J., Lindsay, J., McCrystal, P., & Baidoun, N. (2006). The impact of political conflict on social work: Experiences from Northern Ireland, Israel and Palestine. *British Journal of Social Work*, *36*(3), 435–450. doi:10.1093/bjsw/bcl009

Reed, R. V., Fazel, M., Jones, L., Panter-Brick, C., & Stein, A. (2012). Mental health of displaced and refugee children resettled in middle- and low-income countries: Risk and protective factors. *The Lancet*, *379*(9812), 250–265. doi:10.1016/S0140-6736(11)60050-0

Rousseau, C., Drapeau, A., & Platt, R. (2004). Family environment and emotional and behavioural symptoms in adolescent Cambodian refugees: Influence of time, gender, and acculturation. *Medicine, Conflict and Survival*, *20*(2), 151–165. doi:10.1080/1362369042000234735

Rousseau, C., Mekki-Berrada, A., & Moreau, S. (2001). Trauma and extended separation from family among Latin American and African refugees in Montreal. *Psychiatry: Interpersonal & Biological Processes*, *64*(1), 40–59. doi:10.1521/psyc.64.1.40.18238

Shakya, Y. B., Guruge, S., Hynie, M., Htoo, S., Akbari, A., Jandu, B. B., … Forster, J. (2014). Newcomer refugee youth as 'resettlement champions' for their families: Vulnerability, resilience and empowerment. In L. Simich & L. Andermann (Eds.), *Refuge and Resilience* (pp. 131–154). New York, NY: Springer.

Stewart, J. (2011). *Supporting refugee children: Strategies for educators*. Toronto, Ontario: University of Toronto Press.

Thomson, M. J. (2017). Revoked: Refugee bans in effect. In D. Haines, J. Howell, & F. Keles (Eds.), *Maintaining refuge: Anthropological reflections in uncertain times* (pp. 95–104). New York Chichester, West Sussex: American Anthropological Association: A Publication of the Committee on Refugees and Immigrants.

UNHCR. (2017a). *Global trends: Forced displacement in 2016*. Geneva, Switzerland: Author. Retrieved from http://www.unhcr.org/5943e8a34.pdf

UNHCR. (2017b, April 24). *Canada's 2016 record high level of resettlement praised by UNHCR*. Geneva, Switzerland: Author. Retrieved from http://www.unhcr.org/news/press/2017/4/58fe15464/canadas-2016-record-high-level-resettlement-praised-unhcr.html

UNHCR. (2018). *US refugee resettlement facts: January 2018*. Geneva, Switzerland: Author. Retrieved from http://www.unhcr.org/us-refugee-resettlement-facts.html

UNICEF., United Nations. Office of the Special Representative of the Secretary-General for Children, & Armed Conflict. (2009). *Machel study 10-year strategic review: Children and conflict in a changing world*. New York, NY: UNICEF.

Vasudevan, L. (2011). An invitation to unknowing. *Teachers College Record, 113*(6), 1154–1174.

Werner, E. E. (2012). Children and war: Risk, resilience, and recovery. *Development and Psychopathology, 24*(2), 553–558. doi:10.1017/S0954579412000156

Wessells, M. (2002). Recruitment of children as soldiers in sub-Saharan Africa: An ecological analysis. In Mjøset, L., & Van Holde, S. (Eds.), *The comparative study of conscription in the armed forces* (pp. 237–254). Emerald Group Publishing Limited.

Williams, R., & Drury, J. (2011). Personal and collective psychosocial resilience: Implications for children, young people and their families involved in war and disasters. In Cook, D., & Wall, J. (Eds.), *Children and armed conflict: Cross-disciplinary investigations* (pp. 57–75). London: Palgrave Macmillan.

Wilson, R. M., Murtaza, R., & Shakya, Y. B. (2010). Pre-migration and post-migrationdeterminants of mental health for newly arrived refugees in Toronto. *Canadian Issues: Immigrant Mental Health, Summer*, 45–50.

Woodford, M. A. (2006). Family: Non-traditional. In F. J. Turner (Ed.), *Encyclopedia of Canadian social work* (pp. 136–137). Waterloo, Ontario: Wilfrid Laurier Univ. Press.

Yan, M. C., & Anucha, U. (2017). *Working with immigrants and refugees: Issues, theories, and approaches for social work and human service practice*. Oxford, England: Oxford University Press.

Zong, J., & Batalova, J. (2015). Refugees and asylees in the United States. *Migration Policy Institute, 28*. Retrieved from http://www.migrationpolicy.org/article/refugees-and-asylees-united-states

Intergenerational resilience in families affected by war, displacement, and migration: "It runs in the family"

Myriam Denov, Maya Fennig, Marjorie Aude Rabiau, and Meaghan C. Shevell

ABSTRACT

This article argues for an expansion of the focus on resilience as a characteristic of the individual to one of resilience as a familial and intergenerational experience. Drawing upon a case study of a young person's tumultuous journey from war to refuge, the authors explore the impact, challenges, and opportunities inherent within the context of war-induced flight, migration, and resettlement, with special attention to individual, family and intergenerational resilience. The authors demonstrate that in the face of adversity and loss, war-affected families do not only run from war, but are also able to repair, grow, and even pass down their adaptive capacities from the "recovery repertoire" to the next generation. Given the capacity for intergenerational resilience, it is the authors' contention that interventions and practices aimed to support the psychosocial well-being of war-affected children must therefore consider the prominence of not only daily stressors, but also protective factors at each level of youth's socioecological system to bolster resilience. Additionally, we argue that social work practice and interventions must broaden service options to include attention to caregiver mental health along with the mental health of the war-affected child to capture the complexities of the intergenerational transmission of both trauma and resilience.

Understanding war-induced migration: realities and implications

Exposure to wartime violence has been shown to be a key risk factor on children's[1] psychological functioning (Fazel, Reed, Panter-Brick, & Stein, 2012). The increase in armed conflict in countries like Syria, Democratic Republic of the Congo, Iraq, South Sudan, and Afghanistan represents the highest level of human suffering since World War II where children are killed, injured, orphaned, separated from family, and/or recruited into armed groups. War ruptures the fabric of life that supports healthy child development, causes injury and illness, severs familial and social networks, and breaks down the structures that provide preventive, curative, and ameliorative care (Devakumar, Birch, Osrin, Sondorp, & Wells, 2014). Although most modern wars are short lived and occur within national boundaries, others are protracted, continuing for decades and affecting multiple generations. In addition, the United Nations estimates that more than 60 million people worldwide are currently displaced by war, armed conflict, or persecution. In 2016 alone, 3.2 million people were displaced, the leading source countries being Syria and South Sudan (UNHCR, 2016a). In fact, flight as a result of armed conflict is at a 20-year high, whereas the number of internally displaced persons is at its highest level in 50 years (Miller & Rasmussen, 2017). Children comprise 52% of the 60 million forcibly displaced by war worldwide (UNHCR, 2016b).

Direct experiences of war and armed violence are not the only challenges to the health and well-being of war-affected populations. Children and families who flee violence and persecution and resettle in other countries often endure great psychosocial challenges during displacement and continue to suffer challenges after their arrival in a new context (Fazel et al., 2012). Research has consistently shown that the mental health impact of armed conflict is either compounded or alleviated by contexts of migration and resettlement. In this sense, "the mental health of refugees is powerfully influenced by war-related violence and loss *combined with* the conditions they encounter en route to, and within, their host countries" (Miller & Rasmussen, 2017, p. 129). Given this reality, it is vital to understand the context and realities of war-induced flight, migration, and resettlement, as well as their subsequent implications for the well-being of these children and families on the run.

In terms of flight, as a result of war, more than 80% of refugees are displaced internally or have fled across national border to neighbouring countries, the majority being located in low- and lower middle-income countries. However, war-induced migration is seldom a situation where an individual or family travels from their country of origin directly to a host country. Far from a linear pathway from the country of origin to the eventual site of permanent resettlement, flight is often protracted, convoluted, and highly insecure. As an example, 13 million Syrians have been displaced by the war, the majority to neighboring countries. Lebanon, a small country of 4.5 million persons now accommodates as many Syrian refugees as the whole of Europe (Silove, Ventevogel, & Rees, 2017). Syrian children and families are living in situations of insecurity and at risk of violence, abuse, sexual exploitation, trafficking, decreased livelihood opportunities, and recruitment into gangs and commercial sexual exploitation (UNHCR, 2013; Usta & Masterson, 2015). Additionally, 314,000 people remain displaced from Darfur in Eastern Chad, and more than one million Somalis live as displaced persons in Kenya, Ethiopia, Djibouti, and Yemen (Silove et al., 2017).

Situations of flight may expose refugees to serious injury, rape, imprisonment, torture, and combat situations (Van Ee, Mooren, & Kleber, 2014). In their study of unaccompanied minors who fled war situations, Denov and

Bryan (2012) highlight the ways in which for refugees, flight frequently involved not only running from violence and warfare, but also profound experiences of famine, drought, traveling on foot long distances. For one half of the world's refugees, flight also means remaining in protracted situations within unstable and insecure contexts, often in refugee camps in deplorable conditions with minimal services and rights (Shakya et al., 2014). As an example, Dadaab, a vast refugee camp in Kenya, has housed families that have been living in this remote and insecure location for more than three generations. Although intended to be places of "refuge," refugee camps are instead places of high insecurity due to food scarcity, violent crime, a lack of policing, and internal conflict related to events extending beyond their borders. These conditions have shown to have a deleterious impact on children's mental health (Rothe et al., 2002).

Although flight presents profound challenges, so does resettlement. As Cohen and Deng (1998) have noted, "Many think of displacement as a temporary problem that disappears upon return home or resettlement…it is often a long-term phenomenon that disrupts the lives of not only the individuals and families concerned but also of whole communities and societies" (p. 23). Indeed, research has shown that postmigration stressors profoundly affect the mental health and well-being for adults and children. In fact, it has been shown that postmigration stressors predict distress as powerfully as war exposure (Miller & Rasmussen, 2017). Postmigration stressors have been shown to worsen the physical and mental health of refugees (Shakya et al., 2014) and include social isolation resulting from loss of social networks (Denov & Bryan, 2014; Priebe et al., 2013), loss of home and homeland (Ee et al., 2013), unemployment due to lack of skill or to host-society restrictions on permission to work (Miller & Rasmussen, 2017), poverty (Rasmussen et al., 2010), perceived discrimination (Denov & Bryan, 2010; Fazel et al., 2012), increased family violence (Betancourt et al., 2012), and challenges navigating uncertain legal status and immigration procedures (Denov & Bryan, 2014; Fazel et al., 2012; Miller & Rasmussen, 2017), to name but a few.

In this article, we argue that with war-induced migration currently on the rise, its familial and intergenerational impact, both positive and negative, deserve far greater attention. To substantiate our argument, we have divided the article into two main parts. First, we summarize recent findings regarding the impact of war, migration, and displacement on family members and the family as a whole. Following this, we draw upon a case study of a young person who migrated to Canada from a war-affected country to explore the impact, challenges, and opportunities inherent within the context of war-induced flight, migration, and resettlement, with special attention to individual, family, and intergenerational realities—particularly as they relate to intergenerational resilience. By drawing upon this case study, we demonstrate that in the face of profound adversity, war-affected families do not only run from war, but also are able to repair, grow, and even pass down their adaptive capacities to the "recovery repertoire" to the next generation. In essence, though the act of physically "running" was a significant and protective theme and strategy for the young person whose life we highlight, during and following war, we show that resilience can also "run in the family," in a powerful intergenerational sense. We conclude with a discussion of the implications for social work practice and the challenges and opportunities in better meeting the unique needs of war-affected children and families.

War, migration, resettlement, and the family

A family perspective

It is vital to recognize that war and migration affect not only individuals, but also the entire family. Families are often displaced from their homes and separated from one another, and the associated emotional stress may impair the ability to provide care and nurturance to young children (Betancourt, McBain, Newnham, & Brennan, 2015). Moreover, mental health issues, affecting a family's ability to function, can persist long after the conflict has ended. As an example, researchers found that symptom rates in those who had suffered from mass violence remained elevated for a decade after the Cambodian conflict (Mollica, McInnes, Poole, & Tor, 1998).

Moreover, family members may experience and respond to war and migration differently, depending upon age, gender, their roles in the family structure, the surrounding context, alongside other intersecting factors. For example, the fallout of conflict, displacement, and resettlement may lead to a transformation in young people's roles and responsibilities (Hampshire et al., 2008), whereby youth take on increased responsibilities and are active in promoting social cohesion and family unity. During resettlement, children typically learn the host language more rapidly than their parents (Birman, 2006). As a result, a "role reversal" may occur whereby it is the children rather than the parents who often speak for the family in negotiating with officials and bureaucracy, thus taking on leadership roles in their family that would normally be taken on by parents. In their study of refugee youth resettlement, Shakya and colleagues (2014) found that refugee youth reported to have the following responsibilities: navigating services, doing interpretation, taking care of family sponsorship applications, earning income, finding housing, sending money back home, mentoring siblings, as well as caretaking responsibilities and giving emotional support. As a result, Shakya et al. (2014) argue that refugee youth are serving as "resettlement champions" for their families in their host country. The authors also show that though refugee youth articulate a sense of self-initiative and empowerment in their new-found roles in resettlement, they are simultaneously concerned about the burdens of these imposed responsibilities.

Conflict-related displacement may lead to changes in gender relations, with women commonly taking on increased economic responsibilities, sometimes resulting in increased power, political participation, and autonomy for women (Hampshire et al., 2008). At the same time, however, Van Ee et al. (2014) note that following resettlement in a new context and environment a mother may feel uncertain about her role and ability to nurture her child-(ren). The reconfiguration of family roles is further complicated in refugee camp settings in which families suffer from prolonged uncertainty and difficult living conditions (Hynie, Guruge, & Shakya, 2013). For example, Hampshire et al. (2008) found that for families living in a refugee camp in Ghana, this reconfiguration led to the blurring of generational categories such as reversals in the life-course chronology (e.g., elders loss of "adult status," autonomy, and authority). Moreover, parenting without a familiar support network and supportive extended family and community may be a complicated task for refugees and asylum seekers, often leading to profound social isolation (Weine et al., 2004).

The longer-term realities of resettlement similarly have a powerful impact on family relationships and family structures. Resettled families may have family still living in their country of origin, as well as scattered across the globe (Weine et al., 2004). Despite having endured significant hardships, once resettled to a new country, refugee populations may find themselves in situations where food insecurity is no longer an issue, and health care, education, and employment are now more accessible. Given their situations relative to those left behind, resettlement and the material security it offers may bring feelings of guilt when considering the situation of their loved ones who continued to suffer (Denov & Bryan, 2014). Remittance and the financial support of family members still in the country of origin is common. Although mitigating some of the guilt associated with resettlement as well as the anxiety concerning the well-being of friends and family, ensuring regular support requires considerable sacrifice and stress (Denov & Bryan, 2014).

Intergenerational transmission of trauma

It is also vital to note that children may be affected by their parents' experiences of war, even if they did not experience war directly. In this sense, children may consciously and unconsciously absorb their parents' experiences of abuse, discrimination, and trauma into their lives. This phenomenon has been referred to as the *"intergenerational transmission of trauma,"* whereby the cumulative effects of trauma are passed down along generations, often amplifying other unpredictable impacts. Evans-Campbell

(2008) puts forward the following definition of the concept of intergenerational trauma:

> A collective complex trauma inflicted on a group of people who share a specific group identity or affiliation – ethnicity, nationality, and religious affiliation. It is the legacy of numerous traumatic events a community experiences over generations and encompasses the psychological and social responses to such events. (p. 320)

Intergenerational trauma was first observed in 1966 by clinicians who were alarmed by the number of children of survivors of the Nazi Holocaust seeking treatment in clinics in Canada (Rakoff, 1966; Rakoff, Sigal, & Epstein, 1966). Clinicians in the United States and Israel, later explored the realities of the "second generation" (Davidson, 1980). Although this was a recognized phenomenon following the Holocaust, it is one that has likely existed across time and contexts. Danieli (1998), a prominent scholar in the study of intergenerational trauma in both theory and practice, wrote:

> Multigenerational transmission of trauma is an integral part of human history. Transmitted in word, writing, body language, and even in silence, it is as old as humankind. It has been thought of, alluded to, written about, and examined in both oral and written histories in all societies, cultures, and religions. (p. 2)

Recently, researchers have turned their attention to the transgenerational effects of trauma on non-Western refugee families. In refugee families affected by war, studies found an association between parents' symptoms of posttraumatic stress disorder (PTSD) and children's psychological difficulties (Betancourt et al., 2015; Panter-Brick, Grimon, & Eggerman, 2014). Moreover, a systematic literature review highlighted that among displaced and refugee children resettled in high-income countries, "some types of parental exposures are more strongly associated with children's mental health problems than are children's own exposures, particularly if parents have been tortured or are missing" (Fazel et al., 2012, p. 271). However, the exact mediating mechanisms responsible for the association between refugee parents' PTSD symptoms and the well-being of their children are still unclear. This has led some researchers to focus on the parent–child interaction as a possible casual pathway, arguing that it is not trauma that is transmitted between generations. "Traumatization can cause parenting limitations, and these limitations disrupt the development of the young child" (van Ee, Kleber & Jongmans, 2016, p. 186).

Indeed, studies focusing on the effects of parental trauma on refugee families have shown that attachment representations (Blankers, 2013), patterns of trauma communication in the family (Dalgaard & Montgomery, 2015), and family violence (Catani, Schauer, & Neuner, 2008; Panter-Brick et al., 2014) have a significant impact on the mental health of children in families affected by war and forced displacement. PTSD symptom severity, which can lead to poorer parenting, has also been proposed as a mediating pathway (Palosaari, Punamaki, Qouta, & Diab, 2013).

Researchers have begun to look at the possibility of offspring inheriting the negative effects of traumatic experiences via molecular memory. It has been argued that parents may actually pass down the consequences of their past experiences to their children in utero via an epigenetic process (Gapp et al., 2014). Findings in this field are inconclusive, yet some preliminary data generated from animal studies and a growing human evidence base has led researchers to suggest that maternal stress and PTSD may confer risk for long-term stress regulation, PTSD, and overall poor mental health in offspring (Yehuda & Bierer, 2009).

Family and intergenerational resilience: thriving together

Resilience in the face of adversity

Although acknowledging the deleterious effect of traumatic stress in recent decades, researchers have begun to shift toward a resilience perspective (Betancourt & Khan, 2008; Southwick, Bonanno, Masten, Panter-Brick, & Yehuda, 2014). These researchers have highlighted that experiences of trauma generate pathology, yet families endure, overcome, and even grow after adverse events (Vogel & Pfefferbaum, 2014). Ungar (2008) defines resilience as follows:

> In the context of exposure to significant adversity, whether psychological, environmental, or both, resilience is both the capacity of individuals to navigate their way to health-sustaining resources, including opportunities to experience feelings of well-being, and a condition of the individual's family, community and culture to provide these health resources and experiences in culturally meaningful ways. (p. 225)

The growing body of literature on resilience and war has highlighted children's and families' abilities to "bounce back," "beat the odds," and "cope well" despite experiences of profound adversity and the presence of individual, familial, and structural stressors (Denov & Akesson, 2017; Fernando & Ferrari, 2013). For example, Klasen and colleagues (2010) have suggested that severe adversity can lead to "posttraumatic growth" or "posttraumatic resilience," terms that describe trauma survivors with a positive posttraumatic mental health outcome.

Moreover, research with war-affected youth highlights the importance of recognizing that the manner which resilience is understood and expressed varies significantly across sociocultural contexts (Tol, Song, & Jordans, 2013; Vindevogel et al., 2015). As such, we cannot simply equate resilience with a set of preexisting attributes because it is often negotiated and driven by culturally and contextually-specific goals and meaning-making processes

(Panter-Brick, 2015). For example, for Nepali former soldiers and Palestinian youth, political affiliation and resistance seems to be a protective factor (Kohrt et al., 2010; Nguyen-Gillham, Giacaman, Naser, & Boyce, 2008), whereas for Bosnian youth the opposite was observed (Jones, 2002). Similarly, Somasundaram and Sivayokan's (2013) study in Sri Lanka, and Panter-Brick's (2015) work in Afghanistan reveal that in contrast to the individualistic views of well-being common in Europe and the US, resilience is often a collective experience, embedded in youth's family and community networks. These examples, as well as many others, highlight that rather than a fixed quality or trait, youth resilience amid war and political conflict is "a complex package of better and poorer functioning that varies over time and in direct relationship to social, economic, and political opportunities" (Barber, 2013, p. 461).

Family resilience

The recent burgeoning literature and reorientation on strengths and capacities has led to an examination of family resilience, exploring the wider relational context of family relationships that promote resilience (Luthar et al., 2000; Patterson, 2002). Rather than understanding resilience as merely a sum of capacities of individual family members, family resilience captures the interplay between individual members and the family unit (Simon, Murphy, & Smith, 2005). Walsh (1996, 2016) has conceptualized family resilience as a dynamic process that draws on the relational resources of the family unit in fostering positive adaptations that mutually support family members in a challenging context. However, it is important to note that resilience is more than surviving, but thriving with the potential for growth (Black & Lobo, 2008; Walsh, 1996; White, Richter, Koeckeritz, Munch, & Walter, 2004). In this way, families cannot only overcome a challenging context together, but also in the process become more resourceful and thus more resilient and resistant to future challenges and disruptions.

In Black and Lobo's (2008) examination of prominent family resilience factors, they found the following characteristics: positive outlook, spirituality, family member accord, flexibility, family communication, financial management, family time, shared recreation, routines and rituals, and a support network. Walsh (1996) argued that a key component of family resilience lies in the "transactional" or relational pathways that families foster coherence, collaboration, competence, and confidence in coping.

Intergenerational transmission of resilience

Although a significant body of research has informed ongoing debates on the intergenerational transmission of trauma, efforts to better understand the intergenerational transmission of resilience are still in their infancy. Currently, there lacks a consistent and explicit definition of *intergenerational resilience*, resulting in variance in the way it has been conceptualized and consequentially the way it has been applied. Similar to trauma research, intergenerational resilience is premised on the theoretical framework of salutogenesis (Antonovsky, 1987), or the ability to overcome challenges, emphasizing the mediating link between parents and offspring. However, efforts to explain intergenerational resilience have largely focused on causal mechanisms or how it can be measured. For example, several authors focus on the makeup of intergenerational resilience, identifying key determinants—similar to identifying protective factors (Field, Muong, & Sochanvimean, 2013; Kazlauskas, Gailiene, Vaskeliene, & Skeryte-Kazlauskiene, 2017; Schofield, Conger, & Neppl, 2014). Existing literature implies that *intergenerational resilience* refers to the process of transmitting resilience across generations (Atallah, 2017). However, a richer and more concrete understanding of the concept itself is still emerging. Rawluk's (2012) examination of indigenous depictions of intergenerational resilience in Canada's Northwest Territories describes intergenerational resilience as a "holistic concept of balance" that brings people together in "an opportunity for intergenerational learning and for honouring the lived experience of each generation" (p. 108). Although focused more on environmental sustainability, the Alliance for Intergenerational Resilience (n.d.) aims to enhance social-ecological resilience by deepening intergenerational connections and balancing different interconnected forces such as elders and youth (Williams & Claxton, 2017).

Similar to the study of the intergenerational transmission of trauma, a majority of the literature on intergenerational resilience has focused on Holocaust survivors and their families (Braga, Mello, & Fiks, 2012; Shmotkin, Shrira, Goldberg, & Palgi, 2011), with only a few studies addressing other war-affected populations. Some exceptions include Kazlauskas and colleagues (2017) who demonstrate a significant relationship between parents surviving political violence in Lithuania and their offspring exhibiting high levels of coherence. Additionally, through a community-based qualitative study (Atallah, 2017), participants developed a conceptual model representing Palestinian Refugee Family Trees of Resilience that demonstrates how families cultivate resilience across generations. Song, Tol, and Jong's (2014) study on former child soldiers and their children in Burundi revealed a local idiom for intergenerational resilience, *Indero Y'umwana Ibazwa Nyina* (*Indero* for short), meaning "education of the child by his mother" and referring to a multidimensional set of values guiding child-rearing. For these former child soldiers, *Indero* took on an added special meaning in cultivating specific coping and survival strategies (and was not present in Burundi civilian population). Similarly, Rawluk, Illasiak, and Parlee (2010) examined Aboriginal resilience across generations, particularly in connection to agency and using resilience as a tool for social change. Drawing from this emerging literature, it remains clear that, though promising, the concept of intergenerational resilience begs further attention, definition, exploration, and application.

We conceptualize intergenerational resilience as positive adaptive capacities or knowledge that has been meaningfully transferred to the "recovery repertoire" of the next generation, equipping and empowering them with vital tools to overcome future adversity. Intergenerational resilience, much like a family heirloom, builds on collective memory fostered within the family system, utilizing familial insights from the past to navigate the future (Williams & Claxton, 2017). It is important to note that our understanding of intergenerational resilience extends beyond physical boundaries to include family that is no longer living or physically present, as may often be the case with war-affected populations.

Social workers and war-affected refugees

The need for a family and intergenerational approach

As demonstrated above, trauma and resilience brought forth by war and armed conflict is a familial and intergenerational experience and thus should be framed and responded to as such. Despite these realities, approaches and interventions for war-affected refugee populations have tended to focus on the individual, rather than the family, and/or the broader community, frequently targeting "children" or "mothers" in isolation (Weine et al., 2008). Moreover, most research in these settings remains focused on descriptive mental health epidemiology and the treatment of individual symptomatology (Tol, Haroz, Hock, & Jordans, 2014). This, in turn, has led to a prolific amount of research, policies, and services focused on the study and treatment PTSD assumed to stem primarily from war exposure (Pacione, Measham, & Rousseau, 2013). The social work profession has been a key player within this current trend, often uncritically importing theories of Western psychology and biomedical psychiatry into its disciplinary toolkit (Fennig & Denov, 2018; Masocha & Simpson, 2011). Although not denying that many refugees may benefit from such individualized therapeutic interventions, scholars have recently called into question the universality of the biomedical approach and its ability to effectively respond to the multifaceted psychosocial pain of war-related violence, torture, discrimination, and loss (Miller & Rassmusen, 2017).

Multiple authors have underscored the importance of considering the impact of multiple interacting factors at each level of refugee youth's socio-ecological system—whether family, school, peer group, or surrounding culture (Akesson et al., 2017; Boothby, 2008; Boothby, Crawford, & Halperin, 2006; Fazel; 2016; Tyrer & Fazel, 2014). This has been expanded to include a consideration of socioecological vulnerability and resilience, particularly in understanding the capabilities of socioecological systems to reduce vulnerability, absorb dramatic shocks, and build capacity for adaptation (Adger et al., 2005). Despite the importance and urgency of these calls there continues to be a heavy emphasis on individual maladaptive conditions (Denov & Akesson, 2017; Miller & Jordan, 2016).

Stories matter: A case example of war, migration, and intergenerational resilience

A case study approach

Health and social care have a long history of translating patient/client stories into the narrative structure of the case report for clinical, educational, and research purposes (Steiner, 2005). For practitioners, stories provide a site to gather crucial information in thinking through treatment decisions and actions (Charon, 2007; Kleinman, 1988). For researchers, stories provide an opportunity to examine the meanings people ascribe to lived experience, while gaining insight into wider social patterns that exist in the social world under study (Eastmond, 2007; Glaser & Strauss, 1967). Stories, however, are not transparent reflections of "truth" but echo and interact with the broader familial, historical, social, cultural political, intersubjective, and personal matrix (Kondrat, 2002). By locating stories in the wider social sphere, they can offer an opportunity to explore how war-affected children's lives are constantly shaped and influenced by the powerful systems and individuals that encircle them (Wessells & Kostelny, 2013).

Given this, we argue that stories matter and, as such, we focus on one case of a war-affected young person—whom we have given the pseudonym David. David was interviewed by Denov in 2010 as part of a study on war-affected young people living in Canada (Denov & Blanchet-Cohen, 2016; Denov & Bryan, 2012). David's case was chosen as it illustrates the powerful implications of individual, family, and intergenerational resilience despite persistent trauma and adversity. Not only did David survive several life-threatening obstacles, but he also cultivated positive adaptations—many of which David attributes directly from his mother—that further strengthened and empowered him to overcome obstacles thereafter. Through this case study, we hope to shine light not only on the realities of war-related trauma, but also importantly on a story of individual, family, and intergenerational resilience despite a deeply traumatic and tumultuous experience of war, flight, migration, and resettlement.

David's story

David was born in a small village in a war-torn country in Africa. His father was killed during the war when he was very young and he was raised by his mother. His mother worked on a farm to provide food. They lived in constant fear of David being recruited as a child soldier and having to hide when the armed groups were close by. At the age of 10, while he was hiding from an armed group, his mother was brutally murdered trying to protect him. After briefly living with a family member, he and other children were abducted by an armed group at school and put on a truck. He narrowly escaped with his life a few hours later by jumping off the truck and running away into the forest while being shot at. He was later smuggled to another African country by a man trying to help him. He was transported in a toolbox in a truck across two countries and eventually dropped off in a big city with only a few dollars, when he was merely age 10. In a new country, David did not speak the language and had to fend for himself.

David lived on the street in extreme poverty and was subjected to ongoing violence from gang groups. Six years later, when he was age 16 years and still living on the street, he boarded a docked ship while scavenging for food, which started moving before he could jump off. He hid in the ship's cargo area for 9 days until he was discovered, at which point the ship members threatened to throw him overboard. In the end, the ship members allowed him to remain onboard if he worked doing odd manual jobs. The ship eventually led him to a Canadian city where he had to navigate a complex immigration system. He had the good fortune of meeting a social worker who took him under his wing and helped him through the long immigration process, during which time he was terrified that he might be sent back to Africa. David began to attend school shortly after he arrived in Canada and graduated high school in 3 years. He is now attending university, is involved in sports, and does volunteer work with youth.

Running from war: trauma and loss in David's story

To appreciate the resilience—or the ability to overcome adversity—demonstrated in David's story, it is necessary to first outline the multiple adversities David faced running from war. David's country of origin endured nearly three decades of near-continuous war and instability. As a result, multiple generations of David's family and community suffered from the impact of war trauma, loss of family, friends, home, and other valued resources. With ongoing violence and destruction in the background, David was born into war. David's father died when he was still a baby, leaving his mother to work very hard to provide for herself and her son while constantly worrying about their safety and the imminent threat of him being recruited as a child soldier. The loss of his father, the well-being of his mother, and the stressors of day-to-day life (e.g., poverty and lack of access to education) adversely affected David's overall health and well-being.

David himself was exposed to war-related trauma as a very young child, as he reported witnessing murders and children losing their limbs to land mines. The most salient war-related trauma for David was when his mother was brutally murdered as he was hiding nearby when he was age 10. Following this was his long-feared abduction by the militia to become a child soldier and having his life threatened.

As described earlier in this article, flight is often protracted, convoluted, and highly insecure, which was certainly the case for David. Between fleeing his country of origin, living on the streets of a neighboring country, and eventually settling in a third country, David faced many challenges over years, during which his safety and life were threatened. From ages 11 to 16, he faced homelessness, severe violence, extreme poverty, and famine. He reported living under a bridge for the entire duration, often beat up by gangs and having to resist being recruited into a criminal lifestyle. He was physically small for his age due to malnutrition, lived in very poor hygiene conditions—not owning shoes or a change of clothes.

The migration process aboard the ship was also highly traumatic, hiding on the ship, enduring starvation, dehydration, not knowing what the crew might do when they found him, and then having to contend with immigration authorities of multiple countries before reaching Canada. David lived with the anxiety and uncertainty about his future and where he might end up, not even having heard of Canada before. Upon arrival to Canada, he was placed in a jail cell—another highly traumatic experience.

Finally, David faced many of the challenges described in the literature regarding resettlement. David did not know how to read, write, or sign his name when he arrived in Canada, nor have any documentation, making navigating the immigration procedures that much more challenging. He also reported that the immigration process was not only administratively challenging but also emotionally challenging, at times feeling that he had to defend his story to migration officials who raised concerns and suspicion regarding his identity and his intentions, despite being a child. Language difficulties were also a hindrance for education and work opportunities leading to financial pressures. Moreover, it is reported that refugees and immigrants often feel guilt regarding family still living in their country of origin, sometimes leading to financial support and remittances, engendering stress and sacrifice. This was the case for David, who despite his limited resources, was sending money back to extended relatives in his country of origin. Finally, in Canada David reported social isolation and also experienced several profound and disturbing instances of racism and discrimination.

"It runs in the family": resilience in David's story

Despite the numerous traumas he experienced, David's story simultaneously demonstrates multiple and powerful instances of individual, family, and intergenerational resilience in the face of repeated adversity at all phases—from war, to flight, to migration, to resettlement. In this section, we draw upon the direct testimony and words of David to highlight his remarkable strength, capacity and power. Furthermore, we draw on David's story to illustrate resilience in war-affected refugees, particularly in exemplifying the concept of intergenerational resilience.

David's story is rife with instances of individual, family, and intergenerational resilience at every step of his life journey. During the war in his country of origin, drawing on the values and wishes explicitly expressed by his mother prior to her death, David actively resisted recruitment as a child soldier. Demonstrating intergenerational resilience, David recalled how he invoked the values and wishes of his mother and integrated them into his daily life:

> I guess my mom never wanted me to join the militia. She would tell me "oh, you never ever join this because they are no good for you or for anybody else." And the fact that I see this myself too. So, whenever they came to the village, I just hid.

Furthermore, David enacted his own personal survival skills to escape when the government militia came to his school to abduct and forcibly recruit students. In a brazen act of bravery and courage, David escaped the life-threatening dangers he was facing. The act of running, became a significant feature and strength in David's life, during and following war:

> I was just really scared.... So after [the truck] stopped. They stopped and they jumped around and went into the little store, this corner store, I guess, I don't know what they're buying, robbing. And in the back of the truck there are 7, maybe 9, 9 guys, and what I did, I asked one of my friends "maybe we should jump from the truck and run." And some of the kids they got scared, and me and a couple of the other guys we jumped off the truck.... And we start running. And they saw us, and they start shooting. But luckily, I guess, we just went our separate ways, different directions. I never looked back, I just kept running, running, running.

Following this heroic escape, David was immediately confronted with additional challenges in determining where he was and where to go to escape the possibility of retaliation and/or rerecruitment efforts. Again, here he used his survival skills to seek out assistance to flee the country and run away from impending threats of recruitment and persecution. On the run, David physically endured an incredibly difficult journey by hiding in a large toolbox to evade detection at roadblocks and checkpoints. Drawing on his enormous strength, imprinted upon him by his mother, David adapted physically and emotionally to navigate the obstacles that he faced all along his road to safety. Then, once in a new country, barely age 11 years, alone, afraid, and overwhelmed by the big city, David found himself having to fight a different kind of war:

> And that's a war I had to face. Because I had come from the real war, people killing each other, and now I faced a different kind of war: learning the language, and living on the street, and dealing with all these gangsters, and obviously, I mean obviously … I mean, personally, I would say that, I don't know if you've been there [name of country] but living there it's a war, you can get killed in like a minute. And so I didn't have where to go, no house, nobody to talk to, and I have $6, I don't know the language, and I'm hungry. I didn't know the things I have to do, but I find myself a place, and I sit down, and that's where I found this bridge connecting the port, I went under the bridge, and there was a little hole, and that was my house from that time, well for the whole time I lived in [country].

Even as a young child, David relied on his own abilities to develop a survival strategy on the streets, including establishing a safe income-generating activity carrying people's luggage at a train station. Moreover, David heavily considered the risks in his surrounding environment and calculated measures to mitigate these risks. Specifically, David strategically chose to live on his own, rather than be part of a group, as he tactically felt that living in a group would entangle him in a dangerous and criminal lifestyle:

> There's no housing there, just boxes, it's awful. Horrible, really. So, I saw myself going to that kind of place, and the people there they're crazy, alcohol drinking, drug using, people, everybody there has a gun even though they live in poverty. While I was there, I witnessed myself lots of maybe 3 or 5 guys getting killed, gun shots so that was, it told me, "no". I went away from this kind of life in [country of origin], so I don't want to deal with it. So… I was like "no, I will be hanging out all by myself."

David's story reveals striking examples of intergenerational resilience. Ultimately, the principles and insight imprinted from his mother, even long after she was no longer physically present in his life, reportedly helped equip David with the necessary tools to cope and adapt positively to the formidable obstacles that challenged him at every step of his journey. His mother's words of wisdom prior to her traumatic death, served as a "resilience repertoire" for David to draw from when faced with unfamiliar obstacles. David reflected on the role and lessons of his mother in saving his life:

> I guess that, I could have gotten into lots of troubles, absolutely, there's no doubt. My mom was a very strong person, and I always say "God bless women.".

> Until today "God bless women.. And she taught me a lot. And the thing that she taught me was that you can never ever steal from anybody, never ask for something, you should never ever put your hands on a woman. Imagine this, a woman who had never been to school, who lived in a small village saying that kind of thing. And those two things helped me a lot living on the street in [country]. If it wasn't for that kind of mentality, that kind of remembering what my mom had told me, I could have really been in trouble.

Following a difficult journey of forced displacement, David encountered an equally adverse experience of migration. However, again, he managed to overcome multiple life-threatening encounters. In an effort to secure food for himself by climbing aboard a docked ship, David hid to evade detection while the ship, to his surprise, began a protracted journey across the world to Canada.

> So, I took that chicken and I start eating, but the moment that I try to get outside to go, to jump out from the ship, the ship started moving. And I was like "Oh what's going to happen now." I was really far from the land, I couldn't really jump out and reach it. So, I thought "you know what, maybe I'm just going to hide in there for a couple of hours," because I didn't know where the ship was going, so I'm just going to hide in here and when it stops I'll get out. So, I ended up going to one of the cargo areas, in one of those archways. So, I went and I hid in there for 9 days.

The sheer act of surviving 9 days living in hiding, in a sustained state of uncertainty, demands an extraordinary amount of emotional and physical resilience (e.g., enduring heat, exhaustion, starvation). However, his resilience was tested further when he was discovered by a crew member and reported to the captain; David was threatened with being thrown overboard due to the financial and legal implications arriving to Canada with a stowaway on board. David managed to evoke empathy from the chief office, influencing his decision to allow David to work on board to earn his keep:

> He said I was causing too much trouble, the money was, I guess he was going to have to pay lots of money [fine] having me there, so he, they, he asked the crew members to tie me up with ropes, and he said I will have to go. (pause) I was crying because I didn't know, saying "help me, help me, help me," and he somehow, the chief officer, he kind of, I don't know, he calmed him down somehow, I guess, and he came by, and he said "I'm going to help you but you're going to have to work so hard for the food that'll give you and everything." So, the next morning, I started working, painting whatever, whatever work they can give me.

Furthermore, David was repeatedly faced with rejection and ambivalence by the immigration representatives of multiple countries. Yet David persisted and continued to attempt to seek refuge at each opportunity, "Yeah, but (pause) Singapore, the immigration officer came in, and they know about, they don't take refugees there. China, they didn't want to talk to me. Japan, they say we don't take refugees anyway."

> Myriam: Did you tell them, "I'd like to declare asylum" – did you know what that meant?
>
> David: I don't think I knew what that meant but I said, you know, "refugee." I guess, after I said that, they knew that I needed help, and they say "we don't do that, son." And then from Japan, we came here, to [Canadian city]. I can't tell you that I knew what Canada was.

Once in Canada, David had to navigate his way through the many hurdles of the immigration system, followed by another long process of resettlement. At only age 16, David's encounter with immigration began with a 24-hour holding in detention. Despite his fear of the unknown, David persisted in completing all the necessary paperwork (a process lasting 6 years without documentation) and defending his case before a judge with the help of his social worker. Although this process was highly complex and convoluted, David quickly acquired new skills to acclimate to the new set of challenges at hand. Utilizing his new skills of reading and writing, David worked diligently to prepare for his citizenship examination to secure his status in Canada:

> I was scared maybe I could be sent back. Because if they wanted to send me back, they could, there's no doubt. I was scared they were going to send me back. And that's why I was scared. And what made me scared, I was thinking "if I go back there, there was no place for me to go there." I believe that the village that I'm from, I don't think it exists no more. Probably it's gone by now, all the houses have been smashed by bullets, the mines and everything. So, I don't think there's anywhere, because mostly everyone just went away, just went away … [In Africa], it's a horrible life to live if you have no house and no family. I mean, if I was going to be homeless, I'd rather be homeless here.

Resettlement in Canada was also riddled with challenges including culture shock and experiences of discrimination. It was a challenge for David to make friends in his new environment as he felt a deep incongruence in perspectives and lived experiences. Here, he actively resisted repeated peer pressure to take on normative teenage acts of rebelling, including drinking and smoking—again drawing on his intergenerational resilience "toolkit" passed down to him by his mother, David recognized that this behavior would result in negative adaptations and further adversity. Additionally, David recalls an incident of racism and discrimination in an encounter with the police. David strategically chose to not resist the police officer and accept the fine and not let the abusive, highly disturbing, racialized slurs infringe on his self-image:

> OK, here is what happened: I was driving and he was like "do you know why you were stopped?" and I was like "no officer." I was with my girlfriend. And he starts asking my girlfriend like "how long had you known this guy? Is he pimping you?"

> The he said "We don't trust 'the N-word,' we don't trust 'the N-word,' they're like dogs" and blah blah blah. I didn't get upset at all. What I wanted to say was "you're an idiot." And then I don't know, whatever, he gave me a ticket.

Finally, following his resettlement in Canada, David illustrates family resilience in finding living family in his country of origin and supporting them through remittances. His financial support to these family members enables them to better absorb potential shocks and overcome obstacles. Furthermore, this example underscores the complexity in flows and networks of family resilience.

Also impressive was David's ability and drive to put his talent and gift for running toward a positive end. Once in Canada, he became involved in track and field, eventually training with a local university coach. David used his running, which had been so critical and life saving in his wartime past, to help him cope with the stress of his complicated refugee determination process, "I tried to keep my mind busy by doing well in school and doing track and field…I did pretty good [at track and field] in my school." Although physically not present in his life, David's mother played an instrumental role in his ability to be resilient in the face of trauma. The values and insight that his mother transferred to him prior to her violent murder not only equipped him with the necessary tools to survive, but also empowered him to thrive under such traumatic and antagonistic conditions. David's story of protracted flight, being perpetually on the run, is an extraordinary example of intergenerational resilience—of utilizing adaptive insights passed down from his mother to transform his experiences of trauma and rewrite his story into a narrative of resilience. David ultimately reflected on what his mother would think of his personal journey:

> I think she'd [mother] be really proud.… I sometimes wish she was somewhere around, so she could see me all grown up, I'm 24, so I could share with her all that I have. I mean, I don't have much, but I wish she was here or somewhere around in this world so I could say "mom, come here" (pause – deep breath). I think she'd be really proud. I mean, she did a really wonderful job to raise me by herself and for whatever she taught me to be, that kind of person.

Discussion and implications for social work practice

David's story is an astonishing story of individual, family, and intergenerational resilience in the face of staggering adversity. Returning to Ungar's (2008) definition of *resilience*, David was able to navigate his way to resources to attain posttraumatic growth. His capacity to trust despite unimaginable hardships and his confidence in his coping abilities and adaptive skills are strong individual resilience factors. The strong values imparted to David by his mother, despite the fact that he lost her so young, were invaluable to him throughout his journey and were important familial and intergenerational resilience factors, demonstrating that resilience can really "run in the family." David was able to draw from the different levels of his socioecological systems to reduce vulnerability and build capacity for adaptation. Attending school was a key factor in David's healthy development. Moreover, becoming a citizen was a very meaningful part of his story providing him with a sense of belonging at higher level of the socioecological system.

Such stories of resilience offer great insight for social work practice by highlighting the importance of using a strength-based model, opening windows of opportunities to support coping and adaptation. It also illustrates that the reconstruction of meaningful lives requires the contextualization of the individual trauma experiences within a broader framework, at the family level and the community level. Social workers can use the lens of resilience within a socioecological framework to promote the inherent strengths of families who have experienced trauma while paying attention to broader community, cultural, and spiritual sources of resilience.

Evaluating risk and protective factors at each level of the socioecological system can provide practitioners a guiding map to reduce vulnerability and absorb trauma in order to build capacity for adaptation. Valuable systematic assessment tools which can assist in this mapping process include the "resilience-oriented genogram" developed by Walsh (2016) and the Transgenerational Trauma and Resilience Genogram (TTRG) developed by Goodman (2013). Similar to the original genogram, it allows practitioners to identify risk factors in the client's family history but also prioritizes a search for protective factors and positive influences (Walsh, 2016). Using the genogram practitioners ask, "Who is – or could be – helpful, supportive, and caring? In what ways might they contribute strengths and resources in a team effort to overcome challenges? How might valued, frayed connections be repaired? Where resources have been lost, how might they be replenished?" (Walsh, 2016, p. 621). Including sources of strength encourages practitioners and clients to shift their attention from a focus on problems and deficits to the validation of each family's potential for positive growth. Attention is also given to community sources of resilience. For example, assisting children with the rapid resolution of asylum claims and facilitating their integration in a safe and stable school environment are extremely important practice goals, as they have been shown to protect against the development of mental health disorders such as PTSD, depression, and anxiety (Fazel et al., 2012). However, it should be stressed that as with other tools developed and used in Western settings, genograms must be culturally and contextually adapted prior to their implementation with war-affected youth. As highlighted by Blanchet, Denov, Bah, Uwababyeyi, and Kagame and Bah (2019), many war-affected young people have lost family members in war, and do not relate with a western view of what constitutes family.

The principles of the socioecological framework can also help social workers facilitate a discussion about broader sources of trauma such as structural violence, systematic marginalization, poverty, racism, and oppressive immigration policies (Miller & Rasmussen, 2017). Practitioners are encouraged to work collaboratively with their clients to identify potential avenues to seek social justice or engage in political action (Fennig & Denov, 2018; Goodman, 2013). Critics of the resilience approach argue that it places the responsibility for survival on the individual and as such encourages us to "accept the necessity of living a life of permanent exposure to endemic dangers." (Evans & Reid, 2013, p. 95). Shifting the emphasis from the personal to the political may, at times, be more effective as it allows to address the roots of adversity (Ruiz-Casares, Guzder, Rousseau, & Kirmayer, 2014).

The growing evidence that trauma and resilience are a familial and intergenerational experience is often not translated to effective interventions for war-affected children and families. Although major donors and humanitarian agencies are increasingly emphasizing resilience in their aid strategies (Scott-Smith, 2018), recent systematic reviews of mental health and psychosocial (MHPSS) programs in low- and middle-income countries found a tendency to prioritize direct individual work with children affected by armed conflict (Betancourt et al., 2013; Jordan et al., 2016) and focus on trauma rather than resilience (Pederson et al, 2015). Focusing solely upon individual and trauma-oriented interventions will only offer one piece, even if a very important piece, of the puzzle and therefore will not provide a holistic picture of individuals' and families' narratives and meaning making while trying to rebuild a life in a host country. Given the powerful impact of intrafamilial and community-level risk factors such as family violence, impaired parenting, and material deprivation on children's mental health, there is an urgent need for MHPSS programs to broaden their target and move beyond the individual child (Miller & Jordan, 2016, Allan, 2015). Moreover, family cohesion, unity, and family relations have been found to be key protective factors among refugee children resettled in high-income countries. These are important processes that can be built upon (Betancourt et al. 2011; Fazel et al., 2012; Qouta, Punamäki, Montgomery, & El Sarraj, 2007). Social workers working with war-affected youth should therefore design services that automatically consider not only the children's needs but the needs of their parents and family (Ruiz-Casares et al., 2015). Family-centered solutions must replace the narrow, individualized deficit-based paradigm of current services and interventions to keep the detrimental consequences of war and resettlement to a minimum (Denov & Fennig, in press).

Researchers and practitioners have highlighted that psychosocial support and services show improved or better mental health outcomes when they are provided to war-affected populations through holistic, culturally grounded, family-based, and community-based approaches (Pedersen et al., 2015). The central role of cultural values, identities, and practices in fostering resilience, hope, and a sense of meaning have been emphasized by multiple scholars (Panter-Brick, 2015; Ruiz-Casares et al., 2014; Tol et al., 2013; Wexler, 2014). Families and local communities can contribute a rich array of cultural resources—including traditions, elders, and community leaders; community processes and tools, such as rituals and ceremonies—to assist in the development of psychosocial assistance (Kostelny, 2006). Because these resources reflect community values, beliefs, and cultural traditions, they give voice to community members and thus are likely to be sustainable and provide meaning.

A multilayered, socioecological approach to service provision should be formulated and implemented—one that builds upon the existing strengths of community-based services (Jordans et al., 2016). An exemplar of a socioecological program is Project Supporting the Health of Immigrant Families and Adolescents (SHIFA), a multitiered school-based program developed to provide mental health care for Somali refugee youth and their families. The project is implemented by an interdisciplinary staff comprising mental health professionals, Somali social workers, teachers, and cultural brokers from the community. It consists of three components of prevention and intervention: (1) broad-based family prevention and resilience-building provided to the entire community; (2) early intervention school-based groups for at-risk students and trainings for teachers to help ensure they understand children's culture and mental health needs; and (3) direct individual intervention for youth. The team has found the approach to be highly effective and report an improvement of mental health and resources amongst children and youth in all tiers (Ellis et al., 2013). These and other innovative programs demonstrate the promise of a holistic approaches and suggest that a possible broadening of focus is in progress.

Conclusion

Running was a recurring and vital theme in David's life. He not only bravely and successfully ran from war, but also used the act of running, through track and field, later in his life as way to build strength, capacity, and a means to cope with stress. Drawing on the metaphor of running, this time in the intergenerational sense, we argue that these capacities can actually "run in the family." In the face of extreme adversity, war-affected children and families are able to not only survive life-threatening dangers, but also build capacities and foster personal growth as a result. In this article, we have attempted to expand the focus on resilience as a characteristic of the individual to one of resilience as a familial and intergenerational experience. The emerging concept of intergenerational resilience offers some important insights into the ways positive adaptive capacities or knowledge can be meaningfully transferred to the recovery repertoire of the next generation, equipping and empowering them with vital tools to overcome future adversity. At the same time, it draws attention to the resilience of the family itself and the intrafamilial processes that foster adaptation and growth.

David's incredible story of resilience joins other narratives of perseverance in demonstrating that for war-affected youth, mental health is determined by not only traumatic experiences of the past, but also by possibilities and hopes for the future (Panter-Brick, 2015). Although David faced unimaginable challenges, he was able to persevere while acquiring new skills to not only help himself but also empower others (or even instill resilience onto others). His experiences and actions echo the profound words of Victor Frankl (1959) in *Man's Search for Meaning*:

> We who lived in concentration camps can remember the men who walked through the huts comforting others, giving away their last piece of bread. They may have been few in number, but they offer sufficient proof that everything can be taken from a man but one thing: the last of human freedoms – to choose one's own attitude in any given set of circumstances – to choose one's own way. (p. 86)

In setting goals to brighten his future, David confirms that in spite of unspeakable hardship, life can be given meaning, and so too can suffering. It is difficult to ignore the symbolism in turning a dire situation of constant flight, or continually running from life-threatening dangers, into a healthy adaptation of running recreationally; David's story demonstrates tremendous physical and psychosocial endurance.

Stories of resilience such as David's offer great insight for social work not only because of their ability to demonstrate the triumph of human spirit, but also because they demonstrate the importance of identifying contextually relevant risk and protective factors at all levels of the child's social ecology. Research with war-affected families shows that "a supportive socio-ecological context is at least as an important – if not more important – determinant of resilience as intra- individual variables" (Tol et al., 2013, p. 456). Interventions and practices aimed to support the psychosocial well-being of war-affected children must therefore consider the prominence of daily stressors and protective factors, as well as broaden service options to include attention to caregiver mental health along with the mental health of the war-affected child. Social workers can work collaboratively with policy makers, mental health agencies, and with war-affected community members themselves to develop multilevel resilience-oriented services rooted in the culture, community and context they live in.

Note

1. The United Nations (UN)*Convention on the Rights of the Child* (United Nations General Assembly, 1989) defines a child as "every human being below 18 years." The UN defines *youth* as "those persons between the ages of 15 and 24 years.

Disclosure statement

No potential conflict of interest was reported by the authors.

References

Adger, W. N., Hughes, T. P., Folke, C., Carpenter, S. R., & Rockström, J. (2005). Social-ecological resilience to coastal disasters. *Science*, *309*(5737), 1036-1039. doi:10.1126/science.1112122

Akesson, B., & Denov, M. (2017). Socio-ecological research methods with children affected by armed conflict: Examples from northern Uganda and Palestine. In M. Denov & B. Akesson (Eds.), *Children affected by armed conflict: Theory, method, and practice* (pp. 139–162). New York, NY: Columbia University Press.

Allan, J. (2015). 'Reconciling the "psycho-social/structural" in social work counselling with refugees', british journal of social work. *45*(6), 1699–716. doi:10.1093/bjsw/bcu051

Alliance for Intergenerational Resilience. (n.d.). Retrieved from: http://intergenresil.com/resil-stories/fergus-cgf.html

Antonovsky, A. (1987). The salutogenic perspective: Toward a new view of health and illness. *Advances, Institute for Advancement of Health*, *4*(1), 47–55.

Atallah, D. G. (2017). A community-based qualitative study of intergenerational resilience with Palestinian refugee families facing structural violence and historical trauma. *Transcultural Psychiatry*, *54*(3), 357–383. doi:10.1177/1363461517706287

Barber, B. K. (2013). Annual Research Review: The experience of youth with political conflict - challenging notions of resilience and encouraging research refinement. *JCPP Journal of Child Psychology and Psychiatry*, *54*(4), 461–473. doi:10.1111/jcpp.12056

Betancourt, T. S., Borisova, I., Williams, T. P., Meyers-Ohki, S. E., Rubin-Smith, J. E., Annan, J., & Kohrt, B. A. (2013). Research Review: Psychosocial adjustment and mental health in former child soldiers - a systematic review of the literature and recommendations for future research. *JCPP Journal of Child Psychology and Psychiatry*, *54*(1), 17–36. doi:10.1111/j.1469-7610.2012.02620.x

Betancourt, T. S., & Khan, K. T. (2008). The mental health of children affected by armed conflict: Protective processes and pathways to resilience. *International Review of Psychiatry*, *20*(3), 317–328. doi:10.1080/09540260802090363

Betancourt, T. S., McBain, R. K., Newnham, E. A., & Brennan, R. T. (2015). The intergenerational impact of war: Longitudinal relationships between caregiver and child mental health in postconflict Sierra Leone. *JCPP Journal of Child Psychology and Psychiatry*, *56*(10), 1101–1107. doi:10.1111/jcpp.12389

Betancourt, T. S., Meyers-Ohki, S., Stulac, S. N., Barrera, A. E., Mushashi, C., & Beardslee, W. R. (2011). Nothing can defeat combined hands (abashize hamwe ntakibananira): protective processes and resilience in rwandan children and families affected by hiv/aids. *Social Science & Medicine*, *73*(5), 693-701. doi:10.1016/j.socscimed.2011.06.053

Betancourt, T. S., Newnham, E. A., Layne, C. M., Kim, S., Steinberg, A. M., Ellis, H., & Birman, D. (2012). Trauma history and psychopathology in war-affected refugee children referred for trauma-related mental health services in the United States. *Journal of Traumatic Stress*, *25*(6), 682–690. doi:10.1002/jts.21749

Birman, D. (2006). Acculturation gap and family adjustment: Findings with Soviet Jewish refugees in the United States and Implications for measurement. *Journal of Cross-Cultural Psychology*, *37*(5), 568–589. doi:10.1177/0022022106290479

Black, K., & Lobo, M. (2008). A conceptual review of family resilience factors. *Journal of Family Nursing, 14*(1), 33–55. doi:10.1177/1074840707312237

Blanchet-Cohen, N., Denov, M., Bah, A., Uwababyeyi, L., and Kagame, J. (2019). Rethinking the meaning of 'family' for war-affected young people: Implications for social work education and practice. *Journal of Family Social Work*, 22, 1.

Blankers, E. (2013). A new generation: How refugee trauma affects parenting and child development. (Unpublished doctoral dissertation). Utretcht University, Utrecht, The Netherlands.

Boothby, N. (2008). Political violence and development: An ecologic approach to children in war zones. *Child and Adolescent Psychiatric Clinics of North America, 17*(3), 497–514. doi:10.1016/j.chc.2008.02.004

Boothby, N., Crawford, J., & Halperin, J. (2006). Mozambique child soldier life outcome study: Lessons learned in rehabilitation and reintegration efforts. *Global Public Health, 1* (1), 87–107. doi:10.1080/17441690500324347

Braga, L. L., Mello, M. F., & Fiks, J. P. (2012). Transgenerational transmission of trauma and resilience: A qualitative study with Brazilian offspring of Holocaust survivors. *BMC Psychiatry, 12*(1), 134. doi:10.1186/1471-244X-12-86

Catani, C., Schauer, E., & Neuner, F. (2008). Beyond individual war trauma: Domestic violence against children in Afghanistan and Sri Lanka. *Journal of Marital and Family Therapy, 34*(2), 165–176. doi:10.1111/j.1752-0606.2008.00062.x

Charon, R. (2007). What to do with stories: The sciences of narrative medicine. *Canadian Family Physician, 53*(8), 1265–1267. Retrieved from https://www.ncbi.nlm.nih.gov/pmc/articles/PMC1949238/

Cohen, R., & Deng, F. M. (1998). *Masses in flight: The global crisis of internal displacement.* Washington, D.C: Brookings Institution Press.

Dalgaard, N. T., & Montgomery, E. (2015). Disclosure and silencing: A systematic review of the literature on patterns of trauma communication in refugee families. *Transcultural Psychiatry, 52*(5), 579–593. doi:10.1177/1363461514568442

Danieli, Y. (ed.). (1998). *International handbook of multigenerational legacies of trauma.* New York, NY: Plenum Press.

Davidson, S. (1980). The clinical effects of massive psychic Trauma in families of holocaust survivors. *Journal of Marital and Family Therapy, 6*(1), 11–21. doi:10.1111/jmft.1980.6.issue-1

Denov, M., & Akesson, B. (2017). Approaches to studying children affected by war: Reflections on theory, method and practice. In M. Denov & B. Akesson (Eds.), *Children affected by armed conflict: Theory, method, and practice* (pp. 1–17). New York, NY: Columbia University Press.

Denov, M., & Blanchet-Cohen, N. (2016). Trajectories of violence and survival: Turnings and adaptations in the lives of two war-affected youth living in Canada. *Peace and Conflict: Journal of Peace Psychology, 22*(3), 236–245. doi:10.1037/pac0000169

Denov, M., & Bryan, C. (2010). Unaccompanied refugee children in Canada: Experiences of flight and resettlement. *Canadian Social Work, 12*(1), 67–75.

Denov, M., & Bryan, C. (2012). Tactical maneuvering and calculated risks: Independent child migrants and the complex terrain of flight. *New Directions for Child and Adolescent Development, 2012*(136), 13–27. doi:10.1002/cad.20008

Denov, M., & Bryan, C. (2014). Social navigation and the resettlement experiences of separated children in Canada. *Refuge, 30*(1), 25–34.

Denov, M., & Fennig, M. (in press). Assessing the rights and realities of war-affected refugee children in Canada. In T. Waldock (Ed.), *The status of children in Canada: A children's right's analysis.* Toronto, Canada: Canadian Scholars Press.

Devakumar, D., Birch, M., Osrin, D., Sondorp, E., & Wells, J. C. (2014). The intergenerational effects of war on the health of children. *BMC Medicine, 12*(1), 57. doi:10.1186/s12916-014-0141-2

Eastmond, M. (2007). Stories as lived experience: Narratives in forced migration research. *Journal of Refugee Studies, 20*(2), 248–264. doi:10.1093/jrs/fem007

Ellis, B. H., Miller, A. B., Abdi, S., Barrett, C., Blood, E. A., & Betancourt, T. S. (2013). Multi-tier mental health program for refugee youth. *Journal of Consulting and Clinical Psychology, 81*(1), 129. doi:10.1037/a0029844

Evans, B., & Reid, J. (2013). Dangerously exposed: The life and death of the resilient subject. *Resilience, 1*(2), 83–98. doi:10.1080/21693293.2013.770703

Evans-Campbell, T. (2008). Historical trauma in American Indian/Native Alaska communities: A multilevel framework for exploring impacts on individuals, families, and communities. *Journal of Interpersonal Violence, 23*(3), 316–338. doi:10.1177/0886260507312290

Fazel, M. (2016). Proactive depression services needed for at-risk populations. *The Lancet. Psychiatry, 3*(1), 6–7. doi:10.1016/S2215-0366(15)00470-8

Fazel, M., Reed, R. V., Panter-Brick, C., & Stein, A. (2012). Mental health of displaced and refugee children resettled in high-income countries: Risk and protective factors. *The Lancet, 379*(9812), 266–282. doi:10.1016/S0140-6736(11)60051-2

Fennig, M., & Denov, M. (2018). Regime of truth: Rethinking the dominance of the bio-medical model in mental health social work with refugee youth. *British Journal of Social Work*. doi:10.1093/bjsw/bcy036

Fernando, C., & Ferrari, M. (Eds.). (2013). *Handbook of resilience in children of war*. New York, NY: Springer Science & Business Media.

Field, N. P., Muong, S., & Sochanvimean, V. (2013). Parental styles in the intergenerational transmission of trauma stemming from the Khmer Rouge regime in Cambodia. *American Journal of Orthopsychiatry, 83*(4), 483–494. doi:10.1111/ajop.12057

Frankl, V. E. (1959). *Man's search for meaning*. Boston, MA: Beacon Press.

Gapp, K., Jawaid, A., Sarkies, P., Bohacek, J., Pelczar, P., Prados, J., … Mansuy, I. M. (2014). Implication of sperm RNAs in transgenerational inheritance of the effects of early trauma in mice. *Nature Neuroscience, 17*(5), 667–669. doi:10.1038/nn.3695

Glaser, B. G., & Strauss, A. L. (1967). The discovery of ground theory: Strategies for qualitativetheory. New Brunswick: Aldine Transaction.

Goodman, R. D. (2013). The transgenerational trauma and resilience genogram. *Counselling Psychology Quarterly, 26*(3–4), 386–405. doi:10.1080/09515070.2013.820172

Hampshire, K., Porter, G., Kilpatrick, K., Kyei, P., Adjaloo, M., & Oppong, G. (2008). Liminal spaces: Changing inter-generational relations among long-term Liberian refugees in Ghana. *Human Organization, 67*(1), 25–36. Retrieved from https://search.proquest.com/docview/201169796?accountid=12339

Hynie, M., Guruge, S., & Shakya, Y. B. (2013). Family relationships of Afghan, Karen and Sudanese Refugee Youth. *Canadian Ethnic Studies, 44*(3), 11–28. doi:10.1353/ces.2013.0011

Jones, L. (2002). Adolescent understandings of political violence and psychological well-being: A qualitative study from Bosnia Herzegovina. *Social Science & Medicine (1982), 55*(8), 1351–1371. doi:10.1016/S0277-9536(01)00275-1

Jordans, M. J., Pigott, H., & Tol, W. A. (2016). Interventions for children affected by armed conflict: A systematic review of mental health and psychosocial support in low- and middle-income Countries. *Current Psychiatry Reports, 18*(1). doi:10.1007/s11920-015-0648-z

Kazlauskas, E., Gailiene, D., Vaskeliene, I., & Skeryte-Kazlauskiene, M. (2017). Intergenerational transmission of resilience? Sense of coherence is associated between

Lithuanian survivors of political violence and their adult offspring. *Frontiers in Psychology, 8*, 1677. doi:10.3389/fpsyg.2017.01677

Klasen, F., Oettingen, G., Daniels, J., Post, M., Hoyer, C., & Adam, H. (2010). Posttraumatic resilience in former ugandan child soldiers. *Child Development, 81*(4), 1096-1113. doi:10.1111/(ISSN)1467-8624

Kleinman, A. (1988). *The illness narratives: Suffering, healing, and the human condition.* New York, NY: Basic books.

Kohrt, B. A., Jordans, M. J., Tol, W. A., Perera, E., Karki, R., Koirala, S., & Upadhaya, N. (2010). Social ecology of child soldiers: Child, family, and community determinants of mental health, psychosocial well-being, and reintegration in Nepal. *Transcultural Psychiatry, 47*, 727–753. doi:10.1177/1363461510381290

Kondrat, M. E. (2002). Actor-centered social work re-visioning "person-in-environment" through a critical theory lens. *Social Work, 47*(4), 435–448.

Kostelny, K. (2006). A culture-based, integrative approach. In N. Boothby, A. Strang, & M. G. Wessells (Eds.), *A world turned upside down: Social ecological approaches to children in war zones* (pp. 19–38). Bloomfield, CT: Kumarian Press.

Luthar, S. S., & Cicchetti, D. (2000). The construct of resilience: Implications for interventions and social policies. *Development and Psychopathology, 12*(4), 857–885.

Masocha, S., & Simpson, M. K. (2011). Xenoracism: Towards a critical understanding of the construction of asylum seekers and its implications for social work practice. *Practice, 23*(1), 5–18. doi:10.1080/09503153.2010.536211

Miller, K. E., & Jordans, Mark J. D. (2016). Determinants of children's mental health in war-torn settings: translating research into action. *Current Psychiatry Reports, 18*(6), 58. doi:10.1007/s11920-016-0692-3

Miller, K. E., & Rasmussen, A. (2017). The mental health of civilians displaced by armed conflict: an ecological model of refugee distress. *Epidemiology and Psychiatric Sciences, 26* (2), 129-138. doi:10.1017/S2045796016000172

Miller, K. E., & Rasmussen, A. (2017). The mental health of civilians displaced by armed conflict: An ecological model of refugee distress. *Epidemiology and Psychiatric Sciences, 26* (2), 129–138. doi:10.1017/S2045796016000172

Mollica, R. F., McInnes, K., Poole, C., & Tor, S. (1998). Dose-effect relationships of trauma to symptoms of depression and post-traumatic stress disorder among Cambodian survivors of mass violence. *The British Journal of Psychiatry, 173*(6), 482–488.

Nguyen-Gillham, V., Giacaman, R., Naser, G., & Boyce, W. (2008). Normalising the abnormal: Palestinianyouth and the contradictions of resilience in protracted conflict. *Health & Social Care in the Community, 16*(3), 291–298. doi:10.1111/j.1365-2524.2008.00767.x

Pacione, L., Measham, T., & Rousseau, C. (2013). Refugee children: Mental health and effective interventions. *Current Psychiatry Reports, 15*(2), 341. doi:10.1007/s11920-012-0341-4

Palosaari, E., Punamaki, R. L., Qouta, S., & Diab, M. (2013). Intergenerational effects of war trauma among Palestinian families mediated via psychological maltreatment. *Child Abuse & Neglect, 37*(11), 955–968. doi:10.1016/j.chiabu.2013.04.006

Panter-Brick, C. (2015). Culture and resilience: Next steps for theory and practice. In L. C. Theron, L. Liebenberg, & M. Ungar (Eds.), *Youth resilience and culture: Commonalities and complexities* (pp. 233–244). New York, NY: Springer.

Panter-Brick, C., Grimon, M.-P., & Eggerman, M. (2014). Caregiverchild mental health: A prospective study in conflict and refugee settings. *Journal of Child Psychology and Psychiatry, 55*(4), 313–327. doi:10.1111/jcpp.12167

Patterson, J. M. (2002). Understanding family resilience. *Journal of Clinical Psychology, 58*(3), 233–246.

Pedersen, D., Kienzler, H., & Guzder, J. (2015). Searching for best practices: A systematic inquiry into the nature of psychosocial interventions aimed at reducing the mental health burden in conflict and postconflict settings. *SAGE Open*, *5*(4), 1–25. doi:10.1177/2158244015615164

Priebe, S., Matanov, A., Barros, H., Canavan, R., Gabor, E., Greacen, T., … Gaddini, A. (2013). Mental health-care provision for marginalized groups across Europe: Findings from the PROMO study. *European Journal of Public Health*, *23*(1), 97–103. doi:10.1093/eurpub/ckr214

Qouta, S., Punamäki, R. L., Montgomery, E., & El Sarraj, E. (2007). Predictors of psychological distress and positive resources among Palestinian adolescents: Trauma, child, and mothering characteristics. *Child Abuse & Neglect*, *31*(7), 699–717. doi:10.1016/j.chiabu.2005.07.007

Rakoff, V. A. (1966). Long-term effects of the concentration camp experience. *Viewpoints: Labor Zionist Movement of Canada*, *I*, 17–22.

Rakoff, V. A., Sigal, J. J., & Epstein, N. B. (1966). Children and families of concentration camp survivors. *Canada's Mental Health*, *14*, 24–26.

Rasmussen, A., Nguyen, L., Wilkinson, J., Vundla, S., Raghavan, S., Miller, K. E., & Keller, A. S. (2010). Rates and impact of trauma and current stressors among darfuri refugees in eastern chad. *American Journal of Orthopsychiatry*, *80*(2), 227–236. doi:10.1111/j.1939-0025.2010.01026.x

Rawluk, A. J. (2012). Intergenerational resilience in Aklavik, NT–exploring conceptualizations, variables, and change across generations. (Doctoral dissertation, University of Alberta).

Rawluk, A. J., Illasiak, V., & Parlee, B. (2010). Intergenerational resilience in Aklavik, NWT. In Conference: Capturing the Complexity of the Commons, North American Regional Meeting of the International Association for the Study of the Commons, Arizona State University, Tempe, AZ, Sept. 3-Oct (Vol. 2, p. 2010).

Rothe, E. M., Lewis, J., Castillo-Matos, H., Martinez, O., Busquets, R., & Martinez, I. (2002). Posttraumatic stress disorder among Cuban children and adolescents after release from a refugee camp. *Psychiatric Services*, *53*(8), 970–976. doi:10.1176/appi.ps.53.8.970

Ruiz-Casares, M., Kolyn, L., Sullivan, R., & Rousseau, C. (2015). Parenting adolescents from ethno-cultural backgrounds: A scan of community-based programs in Canada for the promotion of adolescent mental health. Children and outh Services Review, 53, 10-16.

Ruiz-Casares, M., Guzder, J., Rousseau, C., & Kirmayer, L. J. (2014). Cultural roots of well-being and resilience in child mental health. In A. Ben-Arieh, F. Casas, I. Frønes, & J. E. Korbin (Eds.), *Handbook of child well-being* (pp. 2379–2407). New York, NY: Springer.

Schofield, T. J., Conger, R. D., & Neppl, T. K. (2014). Positive parenting, beliefs about parental efficacy, and active coping: Three sources of intergenerational resilience. *Journal of Family Psychology*, *28*(6), 973. doi:10.1037/fam0000024

Scott-Smith, T. (2018). Paradoxes of resilience: A review of the world disasters report 2016. *DECH Development and Change*, *49*(2), 662–677. doi:10.1111/dech.2018.49.issue-2

Shakya, Y. B., Guruge, S., Hynie, M., Htoo, S., Akbari, A., Jandu, B. B., … Forster, J. (2014). Newcomer refugee youth as 'resettlement champions' for their families: Vulnerability, resilience and empowerment. In L. Simich & L. Andermann (Eds.), *Refuge and resilience: Promoting resilience and mental health among resettled refugees and forced migrants* (pp. 131–154). New York, NY: Springer.

Shmotkin, D., Shrira, A., Goldberg, S. C., & Palgi, Y. (2011). Resilience and vulnerability among aging Holocaust survivors and their families: An intergenerational overview. *Journal of Intergenerational Relationships*, *9*(1), 7–21. doi:10.1080/15350770.2011.544202

Silove, D., Ventevogel, P., & Rees, S. (2017). The contemporary refugee crisis: An overview of mental health challenges. *World Psychiatry: Official Journal of the World Psychiatric Association*, *16*(2), 130–139. doi:10.1002/wps.v16.2

Simon, J. B., Murphy, J. J., & Smith, S. M. (2005). Understanding and fostering family resilience. *The Family Journal*, *13*(4), 427–436. doi:10.1177/1066480705278724

Somasundaram, D., & Sivayokan, S. (2013). Rebuilding community resilience in a post-war context: Developing insight and recommendations - a qualitative study in Northern Sri Lanka. *International Journal of Mental Health Systems*, *7*(1), 3. doi:10.1186/1752-4458-7-3

Song, S. J., Tol, W., & Jong, J. (2014). Indero: Intergenerational trauma and resilience between Burundian former child soldiers and their children. *Family Process*, *53*(2), 239–251. doi:10.1111/famp.12071

Southwick, S. M., Bonanno, G. A., Masten, A. S., Panter-Brick, C., & Yehuda, R. (2014). Resilience definitions, theory, and challenges: Interdisciplinary perspectives. *European Journal of Psychotraumatology*, *5*(1), 25338. doi:10.3402/ejpt.v5.25338

Steiner, J. F. (2005). The use of stories in clinical research and health policy. *Jama*, *294*(22), 2901–2904. doi:10.1001/jama.294.22.2901

Tol, W. A., Haroz, E. E., Hock, J. C., & Jordans, M. J. D. (2014). Ecological perspective on trauma and resilience in children affected by armed conflict. In R. Pat- Horenczyk, D. Borm, & J. M. Vogel (Eds.), *Helping children cope with trauma* (pp. 193–209). East Sussex, Uk: Routledge.

Tol, W. A., Song, S., & Jordans, M. J. D. (2013). Annual research review: Resilience and mental health in children and adolescents living in areas of armed conflict - a systematic review of findings in low- and middle-income countries. *JCPP Journal of Child Psychology and Psychiatry*, *54*(4), 445–460. doi:10.1111/jcpp.12053

Tyrer, R. A., & Fazel, M. (2014). School and community-based interventions for refugee and asylum seeking children: A systematic review. *PLoS ONE*, *9*(2). doi:10.1371/journal.pone.0089359

Ungar, M. (2008). Resilience across cultures. *The British Journal of Social Work*, *38*(2), 218–235. doi:10.1093/bjsw/bcl343

UNHCR (2013). The future of Syria: Refugee children in crisis. Retrieved from http://www.unhcr.org/media-futureofsyria/

UNHCR. (2016a). *Global trends report: World at war*. New York, NY: United Nations High Commissioner for Refugees.

UNHCR. (2016b). *Forced displacement 2015*. New York, NY: United High Commissioner for Refugees.

United Nations General Assembly, Convention on the Rights of the Child, 20 November (1989), United Nations, Treaty Series, vol. 1577, p. 3.

Usta, J., & Masterson, A. R. (2015). Women and health in refugee settings: The case of displaced syrian women in Lebanon. In J. Usta & A. R. Masterson (Eds.), *Gender-based violence* (pp. 119–143). New York, NY: Springer.

van Ee, E., Kleber, R. J., & Jongmans, M. J. (2016). Relational Patterns Between Caregivers With PTSD and Their Nonexposed Children: A Review. *Trauma, Violence, & Abuse*, *17*(2), 186–203. https://doi.org/10.1177/1524838015584355

Van Ee, E., Mooren, T., & Kleber, R. J. (2014). Broken mirrors. In R. Pat-Horenczyk, D. Brom, & J. M. Vogel (Eds.), *Helping children cope with trauma: Individual, family and community perspectives* (pp. 146–162). New York, NY: Routledge.

Van Ee, E, Sleijpen, M, Kleber, R. J, & Jongmans, M. J. (2013). father-involvement in a refugee sample: relations between posttraumatic stress and caregiving. *Family Process*, *52* (4), 723-735. doi:10.1111/famp.12045

Vindevogel, S., Ager, A., Schiltz, J., Broekaert, E., & Derluyn, I. (2015). Toward a culturally sensitive conceptualization of resilience: Participatory research with war-affected communities in northern Uganda. *Transcultural Psychiatry, 52*(3), 396–416. doi:10.1177/1363461514565852

Vogel, J. M., & Pfefferbaum, B. (2014). Family resilience after disasters and terrorism: Examining the concept. In R. Pat-Horenczyk, D. Brom, & J. Vogel(Eds.), *Helping children cope with trauma: Individual, family and community perspectives* (pp. 81–100). New York: Routledge/Taylor & Francis Group.

Walsh, F. (1996). The concept of family resilience: Crisis and Challenge. *Family Process, 35*, 261–281. doi:10.1111/famp.1996.35.issue-3

Walsh, F. (2016). Applying a family resilience framework in training, practice, and research: mastering the art of the possible. *Family Process, 55*(4), 616–632. doi:10.1111/famp.12260

Weine, S., Kulauzovic, Y., Klebic, A., Besic, S., Mujagic, A., Muzurovic, J., … Rolland, J. (2008). Evaluating a multiple-family group access intervention for refugees with PTSD. *Journal of Marital and Family Therapy, 34*(2), 149–164. doi:10.1111/j.1752-0606.2008.00061.x

Weine, S., Muzurovic, N., Kulauzovic, Y., Besic, S., Lezic, A., Mujagic, A., … Pavkovic, I. (2004). Family consequences of refugee trauma. *Family Process, 43*(2), 147–160.

Wessells, M., & Kostelny, K. (2013). Child friendly spaces: Toward a grounded, community-based approach for strengthening child protection practice in humanitarian crises: Natural helpers play a critical role in ensuring children's safety during and in the aftermath of crises. *Child Abuse & Neglect: Supplement, 37*, 29–40. doi:10.1016/j.chiabu.2013.10.030

Wexler, L. (2014). Looking across three generations of Alaska Natives to explore how culture fosters indigenous resilience. *Transcultural Psychiatry, 51*(1), 73–92. doi:10.1177/1363461513497417

White, N., Richter, J., Koeckeritz, J., Munch, K., & Walter, P. (2004). "Going forward": Family resiliency in patients on hemodialysis. *Journal of Family Nursing, 10*(3), 357–378. doi:10.1177/1074840704267163

Williams, L., & Claxton, N. (2017). Re-cultivating intergenerational resilience: Possibilities for scaling DEEP through disruptive pedagogies of decolonization and reconciliation. *Canadian Journal of Environmental Education: Special Issue on Activism and Environmental Education, 22*, 60–81.

Yehuda, R., & Bierer, L. M. (2009). The relevance of epigenetics to PTSD: Implications for the DSM-V. *Journal of Traumatic Stress, 22*(5), 427–434. doi:10.1002/jts.20448

Rethinking the meaning of "family" for war-affected young people: implications for social work education

Natasha Blanchet-Cohen, Myriam Denov, Alusine Bah, Léontine Uwababyeyi, and Jean Kagame

ABSTRACT
This article examines how the experiences and realities of young people affected by war challenge the "typical" portrayal of *family* in social work education. Using aspects of duoethnography as a method of inquiry, the authors discuss war-affected social work students' experience of elements of their curriculum and training. The discomforts shared point to important tensions and discords with prevailing traditional social work teaching concepts and approaches. War-affected young people feel that their realities often do not correspond to Western theories of human and child development and resettlement expectations. In making social work education more relevant and useful, there is a need to rethink the portrayal of *family* as well as teaching strategies. As part of this process, an increased sensitivity among social work educators is paramount, not only to the cultural, religious, geopolitically and ethnically diverse realities of children and families, but also to engaging young people directly in the learning process.

Introduction

The influx of war-affected child refugees and asylum seekers from diverse countries who arrive alone or accompanied by parents or caregivers has implications for all aspects of human services, including social work education. The fact that children make up 51% of the 65.3 million forcibly displaced by war worldwide (UNHCR, 2016) require identifying, defining, and providing relevant types of support, which in turn need to be reflected in the training of human service professionals. This questioning and renewal are part of remaining current and ensuring the provision of effective child and family services to a population with increasingly diverse lived experiences.

This article examines how the concept of family in social work education poses challenges in relation to war-affected youth's experiences and realities. Indeed, the idea of the family is central to social work training and practice, prioritized in international conventions and national social policies. The preamble of the *UN Convention on the Rights of the Child* (United Nations, 1989), for instance, contends that the:

> family, as the fundamental group of society and natural environment for the growth and well-being of its members and particularly children, should be afforded the necessary protection and assistance so that it can fully assume its responsibilities within the community. (p. 1)

For war-affected young people whose family life has often been tragically and decisively disrupted as a result of conflict, violence, and persecution in their country of origin, how does one define and portray family in resettlement countries? What are supportive and appropriate theoretical and pedagogical representations of family in social work education?

Issues in conceptualizing family in social work

Prevalent in policies and programming in the Western world is a portrayal of the family as a nuclear entity, historically construed as "permanent, monogamous, married, nuclear, heterosexual, and Christian, and had clearly defined gender roles" (Bala & Bronwich, 2002, p. 148). In Canada, along with other countries in the Global North, social policies and laws have been founded on the basis of understanding the family as the two-parent heterosexual biological model (Bird, 2010). Attachment theories have privileged the mother–child relationship, overemphasizing the role of mothers in caregiving and often overlooking the role of fathers (Thiessen, 2012). Empirical studies with social workers reveal that these dominant perceptions of family prevail in their practice. In the United Kingdom, social workers are shown to have "limited engagement with 'family' as an active, dynamic entity" (Morris, White, Doherty, & Warwick, 2017) with little broader understandings of family. In Greece, social work students depict traditional views on family issues and family roles (Dedotsi & Paraskevopoulou-Kollia, 2015). A study in Israel shows that personal perceptions of social workers' conceptions of family are often traditional, particularly for those who have limited exposure to nontraditional types of families (Gavriel-Fried, Shilo, & Cohen, 2012). Finally, studies in the United States also point toward the need to recognize the plethora of existing family forms, taking issue with the conventional use of what Smith (1993) terms "the Standard North American Family" (SNAF) consisting of a heterosexual husband and wife and their biological children.

The enormous societal changes in our increasingly globalized world require, however, that social workers contend with the transformations of what constitutes family in their practice and education. Indeed, conventional conceptualization of the nuclear family no longer reflects current family realities (Woodford, 2006). And though it may appear that "non-traditional" family forms are "new," many have been "commonplace for decades, particularly in cultures where extended family members are part of the immediate family system, such as among the Inuit" (Woodford, 2006, p. 136). In fact, these "nontraditional" family constructions are arguably more prevalent than actual nuclear families. However, despite the prevalence of the "nontraditional" family, "the nuclear family model seems to retain its privileged status as the benchmark against which other family forms are evaluated" (Okun, as cited in Woodford, 2006). Social workers need to account for the diversity in family life resulting from the rising number of nontraditional forms of living together as a family, changes in gender roles, the growing cultural diversity resulting from increase flows of migration (Euteneuer & Uhlendorff, 2014), and the recognition of Indigenous perspectives on parenting that involve the extended families (Muir & Bohr, 2014). This evolution in thinking about what constitutes *family* is critical because the views held by social workers on the idea of the family affect how they handle or draw up recommendations on key decisions concerning families and children in their care.

Current incongruities between policy, theory and practice mean that social workers often engage in a juggling act. Focus groups in Canada suggest that social workers have to deal with child welfare policy and practice that prioritize more limited conceptions of family—with a particular focus on children and parents for instance—while working collaboratively with clients in ways that reflect an acceptance of diverse understandings of family, the principle of the "best interest of the child" and professional discretionary decisions (Johner & Durst, 2017). Addressing such discrepancies require that social workers be better equipped to think critically of what is traditionally conceived as the "normal family" (Thiessen, 2012).

Along with providing relevant course content regarding diversity as it pertains to race, sexual orientation, ethnicity, and gender, attention is being paid to the pedagogical strategies used for conveying and stimulating cultural awareness and sensitivity. As an example, in the genogram for mapping family systems—a tool widely used in social work education for assessment and intervention (McGoldrick, McGoldrick, Gerson, & Shellenberger, 1999)—some advocate the relevance of a cultural genogram to promote the cultural awareness and sensitivity. As an educational tool used in the classroom, the cultural genogram involves a three-stage procedure that has an individual and group component (Warde, 2012). While stimulating thinking about cultural values, the adapted tool remains biased toward a Western view of what constitutes family. This may be particularly problematic for those students whose "family system is characterized by large fictive kinship or tribal networks" (Warde, 2012, p. 584). Indeed, such examples show the need for social work education to create the spaces for dialogue and co-creation, challenging the notion of the social work professor as the main keeper of knowledge who delivers content unidirectionally to students. The use of arts and creative expressions has been heralded as valuable in providing spaces for students to colearn and support social justice and diversity (Foels & Bethel, 2018).

This article challenges traditional conceptualizations of the family with specific attention to the particularly impact on war-affected students, future practitioners and/or clients. Based on the experiences of current war-affected social work students, this article discusses (1) the need for an expanded view of the family in curriculum content that accounts for the complex realities of war-affected populations and (2) the need for expanded content and greater cultural safety in curriculum content and teaching, with consideration to potentially harmful impacts on students; and concludes with some implications for social work education.

Understanding the meaning of *family*: considerations for war-affected young people

War, violent displacement, and the death of and separation from relatives affect young people and the functioning and structure of families in profound ways, yet the ways in which war and displacement have affected families has been largely overlooked in social work education and practice. Researchers working in the area of children in adversity have—in the past—tended to centre on children's maladaptive, antisocial behavior in the aftermath of war, as well as negative physical and mental health outcomes and scholarship has often followed suit, though there is now an increased recognition of children's resilience and adaptability (Stark & Wessells, 2013). The social work profession has often applied theories of Western development uncritically (Masocha & Simpson, 2011). The focus has tended to be on the individual, ignoring the family system and/or the broader community (Lacroix & Sabbah, 2011). In relation to war-affected children, these realities run the risk of decontextualizing and detaching refugee children and family's key cultural and social context, potentially fostering othering, inequality, and social exclusion (Fennig & Denov, 2018; Nickerson et al., 2011).

Intervention approaches and practices need to move beyond paradigms of trauma and distress and recognize and build upon war-affected populations capacities (Miller, Kulkarni, & Kushner, 2006). In spite of provisions in the *UN Convention on the Rights of the Child* that children hold fundamental participation rights, scholarly inquiry, and the design of services rarely incorporate child participation (Hilker & Fraser, 2009). Until recently, social science research has been critiqued for contributing to children's marginalization by using methods and approaches that regard them as "objects" of research, rather than active participants (Denov, 2010). With the new sociology of childhood, tangible and significant shifts in the conceptualization of children and childhood have occurred whereby children and adolescents are now viewed as social agents able to influence their immediate contexts (Morrow, 2008). Indeed, children and youth possess knowledge and perceptions of their social environment that is valid, and their voices need to be part of the research (Shaw, Brady, & Davey, 2011) to inform practice.

The limited research available with refugee young people sheds light on the complexities of family. For those who resettle with biological family, research shows that the supportive role of the family can be problematic given family instability after resettlement. Although family is portrayed as central to well-being, changing family dynamics can pose a threat to well-being and successful resettlement, constituting a risk and protective factor (McMichael, Gifford, & Correa-Velez, 2011). Refugee parents and children typically face extraordinary challenges upon resettlement, including mental and physical health difficulties, financial stress, and acculturative stressors that threaten positive family cohesion (Pejic, Hess, Miller, & Wille, 2016). For those young people who arrive unaccompanied, marked by forced separation, research shows that they work at connectedness and maintaining a sense of being a family. The configurations of family do however shift, with modes of relatedness not being based on notions of biological kinship but rather membership to a shared community (Coe, Boehm, Reynolds, Hess, & Rae-Espinoza, 2011).

Given the complexities of what constitutes family for children affected by conflict, Ager (2006) offers a framework that focuses on the functional tasks of the family instead of its structure. He contends that in situations of armed conflict, the functions of the family in terms of fostering social access and transmitting cultural knowledge, values, and human capacity are what count. Thus, meeting these functions is central, but how they are achieved will vary depending on the context. In cases where war and armed conflict have disrupted family daily life, these functions will be provided by a wide range of social relationships. Our qualitative research with war-affected youth shows, for instance, that in the absence of formal family structures, all young people reported actively and deliberately developing personal networks that included their peers, surrogate families, and/or communities who provided psychosocial support, information, and/or resources (Blanchet-Cohen & Denov, 2015). As war-affected young people who are now students in social work, how do they experience and feel about the ways the notion of *family* is being portrayed in their educational programs and curriculum? A war-affected student perspective is important, as students who have been caught up in circumstances of war and genocide need to be provided with opportunities to articulate their perspectives, concerns, and needs to inform education and practice, challenging conventional notions of power and what is regarded as "expert knowledge" (Denov, 2010).

Methodology

This article originates from conversations that took place in the participatory axis of our Research Group on Children and Global Adversity. Since 2012, the research group has been working collectively to tackle the theoretical, methodological, and service provision considerations pertinent for war-affected youth in Quebec and Canada, and in particular the implications for policy and practice. Included in the research activities are the formation of a youth forum that operated for 2 years alongside a multidisciplinary adult-led research team (Denov, Blanchet-Cohen, Bah, Uwababyeyi, & Kagame, in press), as well as a qualitative inquiry with 21 war-affected youth (Blanchet-Cohen & Denov, 2015). Although the role and nature of family were not focal points of these inquiries, they emerged as recurring themes of importance that deserved further attention. Participating in the conversation and authors of this article are two engaged academics and three current undergraduate social work students at McGill University who experienced the tragic effects of war and genocide on their families in their home countries.

Initially, our group met to discuss the possibility of writing on the topic of parentless youth in the context of war migration and resettlement. Discussions pointed, however, to the inappropriateness of the wording, causing a discomfort among student members of the team who disagreed with the labeling, stating "I cannot relate to [the term] 'parentless'." This was particularly relevant to one student member who migrated alone to Canada in the aftermath of the war, but his family remains in his country of origin. Although he came to Canada unaccompanied—and continues to live in Canada without family members—as he aptly pointed out, he is not parentless. The conversation led instead to focusing on the way *family* was being portrayed and constructed in their social work classes, as well as some of the challenges and questioning that this raised, alongside their recommendations for improvement. The students were motivated by the opportunity to explain their experiences in light of what they perceived as teaching content or processes that they often perceived as inapplicable and/or insensitive to their realities.

Following this initial discussion, we used aspects of duoethnography (Sawyer & Norris, 2012), which is a collaborative research methodology where researchers co-create narratives to understand how people experience a common phenomenon differently, given their background and past experiences. Duoethnography is not simply an interview between two people; it has a dialogical function as individuals involved search for understanding the phenomenon as they "compare and contrast their experiences" (Sawyer & Norris, 2012, p. 126). The method encourages diversity of thoughts and perspectives "encouraging critical thought, not alignment" (p. 16). Although generally written up like a script where the participant(s) and researcher are the characters, this article presents excerpts from the interviews according to points of conversation that relate to (1) tensions and discords felt as it relates to the portrayal of family in classes, (2) experiences of discomfort as reflected in class concepts or assignments, and (3) reflections on shifts needed to promote openness and diversity in social work education.

Pseudonyms are used in the citations to maintain a degree of confidentiality, given that the students are currently studying.

In terms of process, there were three collective conversations involving the entire team and three one-on-one conversations between the students. The latter were informed by a set of questions that were broad and specific, such as, "Do you identify with the way the 'family' is presented in your social work education to date? How does the current notion of family being used in class reflect your lived realities?' Some questions probed for specifics, such as, When you reflect back on your courses in social work, can you give me some specific examples of concepts or assignments where you felt the concept of family was not well-suited to your reality?" Some questions sought more their perspectives on views for the future, such as, "If you had a message for professors teaching social work, what would it be? What would you recommend?" Students transcribed a conversation, other than their own, which later served as a basis for informing the findings of the article.

Findings

Tensions and discords in the portrayal of the family

All student members of our writing team, who were all survivors of war and/or genocide and had lost key family members, reflected on the gap between the portrayal of family in their social work education classes, and their own experiences of family. The nuclear and biological family were reported as predominant in their courses, which was at odds with their own much broader understandings of family as being based on connectedness, shared culture, location or experience. Students spoke to the contrasts as follows:

Mary: Listen, in my social work classes, family is portrayed as "father, mother and siblings" while in my lived experiences, family is more than that. Family is neighbors, friends like the whole village is my family. So, it's really different.

John: Well for me I think, yeah, I have to be honest with you. I come from Africa, and I come from a tribe, so, family to me in the context of my beliefs in my culture is anyone that I feel has any relationship with me. For example, my neighbors are considered my family, the people that will live in the same village are my family and people that you know – elderly people even though we have no relationship – but because they are elderly people in my culture, they are family.

David: I think that the way family is portrayed in my social work is totally different because of my past experience. It is different because here family is parents' mom and dad … whatever and maybe the kids sometimes. But where I was born, I grew up living with friends.

> Family to me is that because that is what I grew up with identifying as family, which makes it hard for me when they try to explain about family because it is different.

Students specified how in the absence of their own biological family, whom they may have lost in conflict or who remained in their country of origin, they have recreated family. Thus, family was not defined by kinship, but rather by its functions, as reflected in the dialogue below:

John: So for me, in the context of being in North America, I do not have a family here but I still have people that I consider family … because now, I don't have anybody here that I used to know back home so what did I do I made friends with people like you, I've known you for five years, I have known David for a year. Others here now I see them as my family people, I portray them as my family. Not necessarily that we are blood-related.

Mary: So, you mean family is something that can be created?

John: You create your own family. You make your own family based on the context in which you fit in, right?

This was similar for David who lost his biological family as a result of a genocide and shared how he has been redefining family based on their functions and characteristics. He explained:

David: Because in my case as I said, family has always been people who have been nice to me, people who cared about me, I have seen those people [in my home country] or even when I got here. I meet people who are very close, those people that I can depend on, it doesn't matter if I met them 10 years ago, two weeks ago as long as they cared about me, I can depend on them they can depend on me then to me that is family and that is it. So I don't think it has changed because even in my past experience I always identified people who cared about me as a family, people that I can rely on, people that I can ask for support.

John: How do you think war impacts family? How does it redefine? Can you give examples?

David: I think war impacts someone because war impacts family and changes the way we define family.… But then when the war happens there were so many kids without parents, they were so many parents without kids. I think it shifted the meaning of family in the way that it became more about who cares about you, who can you depend on not necessarily parents or kids.

Experiences of course content and curriculum

Alongside sharing how the experiences of family differ from the portrayal in classes, the team discussed how the clash between class content and their lived realities made them feel, providing examples of assignments. Team members identified specific assignments that have been problematic for them, particularly the genogram because it is heavily focused on a traditional view of what is family. Students who were asked to create a genogram in the context of their social work classes described their feelings about the process:

John: Both you and I come from countries that have experienced different kinds of war, or affected by war and when you reflect back on your courses in social work can you give some specific examples of concepts or assignments where you felt that oh my God this is completely different from what I think family is or you find it inappropriate and what made you feel frustrated or disappointed. Why?

This student, who lost her entire family in a genocide, explained:

Mary: I will give an example of one assignment which is called genogram which is like a picture of a family and relationships. So, I was given this assignment, and I did not do the assignment because I did not know what to put. You write the names of people, where they are, their birthdates whether they are dead … you have to mention all this information in these small boxes.… To me, it was complicated, and I didn't know what to put because there are no family members to put. I decided not to do that and I talked to my professor and she was ok with that, I had to do something different.

This team member, who also lost his family in a genocide when he was an infant explained his perspective:

David: Basically, in one of my classes we have to do a genogram and then the genogram was like a mapping of your family, your route and everything.… I thought everyone was happy [with the assignment] because they can identify with it. But it was supposed to be about you and your family. But usually people here [in Canada] teachers, students they have a perceived notion that everyone knows their family […] But for someone like me or someone who has lived through the experience of mine, parents died and you have no one left and you don't know if you have siblings or not and I don't even know what happened [to them].

Having to comply with and submit assignments that did not apply to their realities made students feel singled out, excluded, causing discomfort and often unearthing painful memories of the past. The reflections below speak to some of these sentiments:

Mary: How does it make me feel…? Ah it makes me feel like I am different from others. I feel ashamed of not having what other people call "family", and it brings back bad memories.

David: To me I felt offended because like OK the teacher fails to understand not everyone has that privilege knowing their roots or knowing where they come from or knowing their parents, siblings and knowing everyone in their family.

In addition to genograms, social work curriculum and textbook content has been informed by key theorists in human development, including key proponents of attachment theory, Bowlby (1969, 1973, 1980) and Ainsworth (1973). Traditional attachment theory asserts that forming an attachment to a caregiver early in life, with emphasis on the mother, plays a fundamental role in normal child development and the formation of healthy and secure relationships. Conversely, those who do not have the mother caregiver present early in life, be it through separation or loss, may be at risk for developing maladaptive psychosocial behaviours as a result. Metzger, Erdman, and Ng (2010) explain that, as part of attachment, forming this close bond is an "essential component of an individual's mental health and social adaptation" (p. 4). Team members who were learning about attachment theory in the classroom highlighted the lack of emphasis placed on the dynamic aspects of human development, discounting the resiliency of many who have experienced adversity. In the dialogue below, team members discussed this in relation to the theory of attachment, which as presented in their classroom, did not align with their own perspectives and realities:

Mary: Yeah, I also know that in one of the classes what it is called Human Development Across the Lifespan.… Like there is attachment theory. I remember learning this and what they were saying in these readings was different from what I knew growing up surrounded by friends that I called family. So, yeah maybe that's something that has to be revised.

John: What is new? What do you mean? What did you read about attachment theory that is different from what you knew?

Mary: It's like they were saying how if something happens to a child at the age of … I don't remember but because I was trying to take in my personal experience, something happens to me at the age of this but now what's my personal development, what changed was different from what the book said.

John: Basically, yeah, I see what you mean. To cope with that they say, ooh children who grow up in this type of environment, they can end up becoming this type of people, or people who come from this type of environment if you come from a rich family or if you grow up in the type of this and that environment. But you and I are living examples and David that we suffered war, we lost members of our family, but we became a product of society in a positive way.

The last statement speaks to how the team felt that the theory presented and emphasized in their classes reinforced static and decontextualized viewpoints. For young people who have been forced to grow up at an early age, some of the stages of development such as identity crisis in adolescence were also questioned, "You know, some of us at 12 years old we become adults. We survive."

The team was particularly sensitive to the ways that refugees were depicted not as people who come to a new context and host country, adapt and contribute in resettlement countries, but rather as people in need of help, coming from far away and in poverty.

John: But if I listened to what the system said that because you're from this country, you're going through trauma. So the system was trying to prevent me in a way to say, no, you don't fit into our society.... Because a lot of people believe that they can't do anything because they come from that situation. And they believe it because the system wants them to believe it. I don't. I'm different.

Although being in a learner position, the student team challenged predominant conceptions as not only inapplicable but in many ways also demeaning.

Promoting openness and diversity

In response to what was perceived as an inadequate portrayal of families, students provided several recommendations. Generally, centering around a call for more diverse perspectives and ensuring less ethnocentrism. This involved needing to have more course content that was authored by scholars and practitioners from diverse racial, cultural, ethnic, and religious backgrounds:

John: Well, I mean first of all the courses that I'm reading are written by people from Western perspectives based on the western way of defining what family is.... And also here it's a very individualistic society, they think they see you as individual and you have your own right ... but for me they try to generalize that every culture has to be like the western model.... But yeah in the western culture there are a lot of things that really don't fit into my own criteria so to speak. The books that I have read, they are very interesting but taking into consideration the background where I come from they are missing the point in taking into consideration cultural aspects of how other people define family.

The lack of diversity in authorship of course content and material were perceived as problematic for social work not only because war-affected young people do not see themselves reflected in the material, but also because it impacts the approaches being promoted for interventions.

John: The system is very, very culturally biased. They are very ignorant. Because for them it's just – they have this theory, all of our theories, the Western way of – I'm not bashing everyone. Western way of theory – applying to the Western theory, it doesn't apply to some of us … people have to take into consideration people of different cultures when they are making policies, when they are teaching and when you're writing a textbook.

Along with social workers being better equipped in bracketing their own biases and able to consider multiple and divergent perspectives, students considered the broader perspective important to question the status quo.

David: I think that is also like their fault on how social work is taught. People have this idea or preconceived idea everyone should have this privilege and not everyone has that privilege. I think if I should give a message to students or social workers just to be open minded and try to understand the individual not as a collective because the class is made of people from different backgrounds and cultures. Sometimes we are all put into one basket because that is the system, but we are here to change the system. People are different and come from different backgrounds.

A starting place is providing more training in cultural awareness and sensitivity, to being more knowledgeable and accepting of cultural differences, seen as essential in building a respectful relationship with clients.

John: Understand people where they come from. And train people, the people who work in the system have to be trained to help cultural education. Because a lot of people that I have spoken to find these people are culturally ignorant. If you walk into a clinic and you cover your head [with a hijab], already they have some perception about you. It's not to follow a pre-scheduled way of asking questions without understanding the background…. They follow a rigorous thing, instead of saying, look, maybe change this thing.

John: That's right … I … pray and don't have to see a psychologist. Because that makes me who I am. That's what I believe in. But if you want me to see a psychologist who just tells me what he thinks without understanding that I pray because it makes me feel good. It's not going to

> work. No, it's not. I have never seen a psychologist. I have been getting recommendations and I refuse. Never. When I have problem, I pray. It's gone. Because there's no trust [in practitioners].

Some of this can be as simple as being better able to meaningfully listen, and to provide the space for the different viewpoints to be taken into consideration.

> Mary: You cannot know everything but then try to listen, listen to what other people are saying like for example if in your class you mention something, I think I can recommend to other students to listen to you and do their research to gain more knowledge about what you are saying. Not to ignore what you are saying.

And at other times, it may involve stretching their own thinking.

> Mary: Maybe social workers have to think out of the box, they have to see, to know that we students are different in different ways, we have lived different experiences and they have to take that in consideration like professors while they are designing their assignments… to consider that we are different. When they are designing their assignments they have to know that students have different lived experiences and this kind of assignment is not for everyone. Try to change.

The notions of "openness" and "diversity" are often hailed as the most basic, core, and fundamental elements to social work practice and values. However, the fact that current social work students assert that such values are not adequately being addressed within social work curriculum, course content, readings, or reflected in their peer-student body is concerning and begs further attention.

Conclusion and implications for social work education

This collaborative inquiry has highlighted that the prevailing concept of family as portrayed in social work education is often experienced by war-affected students as misaligned and at odds with their realities, experiences, and perspectives. As discussed above, traditional views of the family continue to predominate, alongside human development perspectives that are rooted in Western worldviews. The experiences and feelings shared within the team point not only to the inapplicability of content, but perhaps more importantly, to their negative implications for students. At best, the assignments facilitated feelings of disinterest and a lack of "fit" with their reality. At worst, these traditionally relied upon assignments and theories were experienced as isolating and exclusionary and promoted feelings of discomfort and trauma. The lack of space provided to critically engage with the materials is also important to consider. Students often approached their instructors to explain that they were not able to complete a genogram as required by the assignment. In both cases, the students were given alternate assignments. This example shows a potentially missed opportunity to engage all students in a critical classroom discussion (without calling out the student in question) of the strengths and weaknesses of genograms when working with diverse client groups, and the implications for clients and social workers, alongside the education process as a whole. Moreover, existing genogram textbooks offered to social work students could benefit from further adaptations to include different types of families (beyond more recent revisions that include nonheterosexual unions, single-parent families and other forms of blended families).

Viewed on a more long-term professional level, if particular assignments, concepts, and theories are experienced as demeaning and exclusionary by social work students, what are the implications for future social work practice and the education of future social workers? In moving forward, a few points would be helpful to consider. In terms of the family, there is a need to rethink the meaning that is being given to *family*. As shared above, it is the function of family that is evoked as central, which cannot rely on a narrow definition that is entirely kinship based and centered on a couple that is composed of a man and a woman (Gavriel-Fried et al., 2012). This point is similar to Ager (2006) who identifies that, in situations of conflict, what is perceived of as "family" needs to be redefined. Modern society has also brought about changes in family structure that call for a broadening of the meaning of the family in ways that may not be that dissimilar from what has been evoked in this article but that will require further inquiry. Although there are certainly multiple examples of social work engaging with more diverse conceptualizations of family, this needs to be further contextualized to include more specific attention to war-affected populations.

Related to the previous point, another issue that arises from this inquiry is the need to pay greater attention to pedagogy. Although shifts are underway within the discourse, these have yet to be translated into curriculum and training: it is not only about "what" is taught but "the way" it is taught as well. One is reminded of Freire's (1970) distinction between "banking" and "problem-solving education." In banking, education students are fed with knowledge, whereas in problem-solving education students are critically engaged in the content. The conversations above suggest that greater emphasis on problem-solving education would prepare students to adapt and respond to ongoing changes in the human conditions. Arts and creativity are being promoted as valuable in enabling this type of learning to occur, with the potential of revitalizing social work education (Foels & Bethel, 2018). It is not about the value and importance of the profession of social work but rather in figuring out how it can best support children and young people given global diversity and realities. Also, promising in terms of approach and pedagogy is the notion of cultural safety that, it is argued, is a philosophy that "should be embedded more systematically at individual and institutional levels, and throughout the student lifecycle, as a promising approach for cross-cultural encounters" (Lenette, 2014, p. 117).

The cocreation of learning and education also seems paramount in moving forward. In embarking on this writing project, the two professors proposed that the team embark on a paper addressing parentless war-affected children, migration, and its implications. Our follow-up discussions with students revealed not only issues that were perceived as more pressing to students, but also some of our own faulty thinking on parentless war-affected children. This knowledge exchange and ongoing dialogue, though not always straightforward or without challenges, was vital and essential to mutual learning, building trust, and cocreating knowledge. If more opportunities for students and educators to engage in open, reflective debate were made possible, our profession has the potential for greater innovation and change, while also ensuring student empowerment and voice. Greater accountability needs to be placed on educators, who have the responsibility to ensure not just the education and ongoing learning of their students, but also their safety in the classroom.

Disclosure statement

No potential conflict of interest was reported by the authors.

References

Ager, A. (2006). What is family? The nature and functions of families in times of conflict. In N. Boothby, A., Strang, & M.Wessells (Eds.), *A world turned upside down: Social ecological approaches to children in war zones* (pp. 39–62). Bloomfield, CT: Kumarian Press.

Ainsworth, M. D. S. (1973). The development of infant-mother attachment. In B. Cardwell & H. Ricciuti (Eds.), *Review of child development research* (Vol. 3, pp. 1–94). Chicago, Ilinois: University of Chicago Press.

Bala, N., & Bronwich, R. J. (2002). Context and inclusivity in Canada's evolving definition of the family. *International Journal of Law, Policy and the Family, 16*(2), 145–180. doi:10.1093/lawfam/16.2.145

Bird, A. (2010). Legal parenthood and the recognition of alternative family forms in Canada. *University of New Brunswick Law Journal, 60*, 264–293.

Blanchet-Cohen, N., & Denov, M. (2015). War-affected children's approach to resettlement: Implications for child and family services. *Annals of Anthropological Practice, 39*(2), 120–133. doi:10.1111/napa.2015.39.issue-2

Bowlby, J. (1969). *Attachment and loss: Attachment.* NY, USA: Basic Books.

Bowlby, J. (1973). *Attachment and loss: Separation: Anxiety and anger.* NY, USA: Basic Books.

Bowlby, J. (1980). *Attachment and loss: Loss, sadness and depression.* NY, USA: Basic Books.

Coe, C., Boehm, D. A., Reynolds, R. R., Hess, J. M., & Rae-Espinoza, H. (2011). *Everyday ruptures: Children, youth, and migration in global perspective.* Nashville, Tennessee: Vanderbilt University Press.

Dedotsi, S., & Paraskevopoulou-Kollia, E. (2015). Social work students' conception on roles within the family in Greece. *European Journal of Social Work, 18*(1), 114–128. doi:10.1080/13691457.2014.883366

Denov, M. (2010). *Child soldiers: Sierra Leone's revolutionary united front.* Cambridge: Cambridge University Press.

Denov, M., Blanchet-Cohen, N., Bah, A., Uwababyeyi, L., & Kagame, J. (in press). Co-creating space for voice: Reflections on a participatory research project with war-affected youth in Canada. In I. Berson (Ed.), *Participatory methodologies to elevate children's voice and agency.* Charlotte, NC: Information Age Publishing.

Euteneuer, M., & Uhlendorff, U. (2014). Family concepts -a social pedagogic approach to understanding family development and working with families. *European Journal of Social Work, 17*(5), 702–717. doi:10.1080/13691457.2014.945151

Fennig, M., & Denov, M. (2018). Regime of truth: Rethinking the dominance of the bio-medical model in mental health social work with refugee youth. *British Journal of Social Work.* doi:10.1093/bjsw/bcy036

Foels, L. E., & Bethel, J. C. (2018). Revitalizing social work education using the arts. *Social Work with Groups: A Journal of Community and Clinical Practice, 41*(1–2), 74–88. doi:10.1080/01609513.2016.1258621

Freire, P. (1970). *Pedagogy of the oppressed [Pedagogia do oprimido.English].* Oxford, England: Penguin.

Gavriel-Fried, B., Shilo, G., & Cohen, O. (2012). How do social workers define the concept of family? *British Journal of Social Work, 44*(4), 992–1010. doi:10.1093/bjsw/bcs176

Hilker, L. M., & Fraser, E. (2009). Youth exclusion, violence, conflict and fragile states. *Social Development Direct,* 30.

Johner, R., & Durst, D. (2017). Constructing family from a social work perspective in child welfare: A juggling act at best. *Journal of Comparative Social Work, 12*(1), 1–34. doi:10.31265/jcsw.v12i1.145

Lacroix, M., & Sabbah, C. (2011). Posttraumatic psychological distress and resettlement: The need for a different practice in assisting refugee families. *Journal of Family Social Work, 14*(1), 43–53. doi:10.1080/10522158.2011.523879

Lenette, C. (2014). Teaching cultural diversity in first year human services and social work: The impetus for embedding a cultural safety framework. A practice report. *The International Journal of the First Year in Higher Education, 5*(1), 117–123. doi:10.5204/intjfyhe.v5i1.196

Masocha, S., & Simpson, M. K. (2011). Xenoracism: Towards a critical understanding of the construction of asylum seekers and its implications for social work practice. *Practice, 23*(1), 5–18. doi:10.1080/09503153.2010.536211

McGoldrick, M., McGoldrick, M., Gerson, R., & Shellenberger, S. (1999). *Genograms: Assessment and intervention.* New York, NY: W.W. Norton.

McMichael, C., Gifford, S. M., & Correa-Velez, I. (2011). Negotiating family, navigating resettlement: Family connectedness amongst resettled youth with refugee backgrounds living in Melbourne, Australia. *Journal of Youth Studies, 14*(2), 179–195. doi:10.1080/13676261.2010.506529

Metzger, S., Erdman, P., & Ng, K. M. (2010). Attachment in cultural contexts. In P. Erdman. & K.-M. Ng (Eds.), *Attachment. Expanding the cultural connections* (pp. 3–14). London, UK: Routledge.

Miller, K. E., Kulkarni, M., & Kushner, H. (2006). Beyond trauma-focused psychiatric epidemiology: Bridging research and practice with war-affected populations. *American Journal of Orthopsychiatry, 76*(4), 409–422. doi:10.1037/0002-9432.76.4.409

Morris, K., White, S., Doherty, P., & Warwick, L. (2017). Out of time: Theorizing family in social work practice. *Child & Family Social Work, 22*(S3), 51–60. doi:10.1111/cfs.12257

Morrow, V. (2008). Ethical dilemmas in research with children and young people about their social environments. *Children's Geographies, 6*(1), 49–61. doi:10.1080/14733280701791918

Muir, N., & Bohr, Y. (2014). Contemporary practice of traditional aboriginal child-rearing: A review. *First Peoples Child and Family Review, 9*(1), 66–79.

Nickerson, A., Bryant, R. A., Brooks, R., Steel, Z., Silove, D., & Chen, J. (2011). The familial influence of loss and trauma on refugee mental health: A multilevel path analysis. *Journal of Traumatic Stress, 24*(1), 25–33. doi:10.1002/jts.20608

Pejic, V., Hess, R. S., Miller, G. E., & Wille, A. (2016). Family first: Community-based supports for refugees. *American Journal of Orthopsychiatry, 86*(4), 409–414. doi:10.1037/ort0000189

Sawyer, R. D., & Norris, J. (2012). *Duoethnography.* NY: Oxford University Press.

Shaw, C., Brady, L. M., & Davey, C. (2011). *Guidelines for research with children and young people.* London, UK: National Children's Bureau.

Smith, D. (1993). The standard North American family: SNAF as an ideological code. *Journal of Family Issues, 14*, 50–65. doi:10.1177/0192513X93014001005

Stark, L., & Wessells, M. (2013). The fallacy of the ticking time bomb: Resilience of children formerly recruited into armed forces and groups. In C. Fernando & M. Ferrari (Eds.), *Handbook of resilience in children of war* (pp. 95–106). New York, NY: Springer.

Thiessen, B. (2012). The family models held by social workers and family policy programmes: Critical remarks on gender and class perspectives. *ERIS Web Journal*, 1.

UNHCR. (2016). *Forced displacement in 2015.* UNHCR official webpage. Retrieved August 22, 2016, from http://www.unhcr.org/news/latest/2016/6/5763b65a4/global-forced-displacement-hits-record-high.html

United Nations. (1989). *Convention on the rights of the child*, 20 November 1989. United Nations, Treaty Series. 1577. 3.

Warde, B. (2012). The cultural genogram: Enhancing the cultural competency of social work students. *Social Work Education, 31*(5), 570–586. doi:10.1080/02615479.2011.593623

Woodford, M. A. (2006). Family: Non-traditional. In F. J. Turner (Ed.), Encyclopedia of Canadian social work (pp. 136–137). Ontario, Canada: Wilfrid Laurier Univ. Press.

Beginning at the beginning in social work education: a case for incorporating arts-based approaches to working with war-affected children and their families

Claudia Mitchell, Warren Linds, Myriam Denov, Miranda D'Amico, and Brenda Cleary

ABSTRACT

Building on the growing body of work that recognizes the value of participatory arts-based methods such as drawing, collage, Photovoice, and drama in work with war-affected children and young people and their families, this article asks the question, "How can the findings from practice based interventions become central to the work of preparing social workers who are at the beginning of their professional programs?" As the article highlights, there has been only limited attention in the literature on what these methods might mean for social work education, particularly in relation to family practice and especially in working with war-affected children. What could arts-based family practice with this population look like? The article maps out a framework that draws together two bodies of literature, the literature on the arts in social work education, and literature on the arts and war-affected children and their families. Central to this framework is a set of five pedagogical practices that align well with arts-based methodologies: reflexivity, situating one's self, observation, ethical practice, and taking action. The article concludes that though arts-based methods as central to the social work curricula are not a panacea, "learning by doing" is a promising practice for those starting out in the profession.

Introduction

This article builds on the growing body of work that recognizes the value of participatory arts-based methods such as Photovoice, participatory video, drawing, Image theatre, and storytelling in work with children and youth who have been affected by war. As D'Amico, Denov, Khan, Linds, and Akesson (2016) observe, such methods have been found to be particularly effective in "giving voice" to children and youth through meaningful

---

Color versions of one or more of the figures in the article can be found online at www.tandfonline.com/wfsw.

participation, while offering researchers and practitioners an entry point into gaining insight in relation to understanding the serious issues arising from living within the context of global adversity. War and armed conflict can lead to displacement and separation from families and community involvement and has a significant effect on children and youth's developmental trajectory and well-being (Osofsky & Osofsky, 2018). For a large number of war-affected children and youth involved in various interventions, arts-based methods may allow them to express themselves in a developmentally appropriate, culturally adaptable manner. They also amplify the therapeutic effort of the interventions in a way that reverberates through the family system model and socioecological continuum of social work intervention and practice. The existing research has highlighted that arts-based methods allow children and youth to represent their experiences in contexts of embodied empathy, promote activism and empowerment, and, for the most part, as a successful intervention for children who may have limited vocabulary to express their feelings (Gangi & Barowsky, 2009; Harris, 2007; Moletsane et al., 2007). Jackson (2015) also highlights the ways in which arts-based methods can enable access to the inner self, bringing to light important concerns from individuals that they cannot put into words, thus facilitating possible therapeutic goals.

To date however, there has been a paucity of literature on what these methods might mean for social work education as it relates to the core values of a family approach, especially in working with children and youth affected by armed conflict. Although numerous health interventions in conflict zones are carried out to deal with the daily realities of children and youth facing profound adversity, there is a substantial gap between translating and disseminating these results at the policy and practitioner level (D'Amico et al., 2016) in areas such as social work education and practice. In using participatory arts-based methodologies, social workers can have an emotional response to the subject material as well as a cognitive understanding of the social reality that children and youth living within the context of global adversity experience and the resulting psychosocial adversity they face. Indeed, Foster (2012) argues that arts-based methods fit the "ethos" of social work practice and allows the participants to "facilitate empathy and challenge misconceptions by giving social workers and other professionals working with at risk groups in society insights into aspects of their lived experiences" (p. 533). Thus, this article takes what we term a "beginning at the beginning" approach that seeks to explore the question, "How can arts-based approaches which are particularly effective in working with war affected children and their families be incorporated into social work education—particularly in the context of preparing new social researchers and social workers to work with war-affected children and their families?" In essence, can the findings from practice-based interventions become central to the work of preparing social workers who are at the beginning of their professional programs?

To address this question, the article is divided into four sections. First we offer an overview of participatory arts-based methodologies (What are they? How are they currently being used?) as a way to set the stage. In the next section, we draw together two areas of literature, the arts in social work practice and the arts in working with children, youth, and families. Our intention in bringing these two together is to develop a framework for using arts-based approaches in social work practice in relation to working with war-affected children and their families. Next we map out what we describe as a set of pedagogical features in using the arts in social work practice with war-affected children and their families. In the conclusion and reflecting forward section, we consider some of the implications of this work for professional development.

Participatory arts-based methods

Previous work has identified and outlined the potential of such arts-based approaches as Photovoice, participatory video, digital storytelling, drawing, painting and mapmaking, and Image theatre to operate as method and intervention that simultaneously seek to empower and actively engage children and youth affected by war (D'Amico et al., 2016). For example, Photovoice (giving cameras to participants and giving them opportunities to work with their own photographs) has been used with children and youth is a way for the participants to identify through photography features of their community that are of importance to them along with situations that need to be changed. By engaging in Photovoice, children and youth reflect in their own way their community's resilience and challenges. Taking photographs and developing captions for these photographs promotes critical dialogue about the important issues in the community by representing and disseminating the photographs and/or exhibiting them, Photovoice aims to reach those who have the power to implement structural changes in the community such as policy makers (Wang & Burris, 1997). Photovoice empowers marginalized youth and "groups of people who do not normally get to speak" (Mitchell, 2011, p. 51) and "has been documented as a powerful tool to engage communities to enable a deeper understanding of the lives of marginalized youth" (Burke, as cited in D'Amico et al., 2016, p. 531). Of relevance to this article, Photovoice has been found to be particularly valuable in work with novice social workers in relation to developing critical reflection skills and in addressing issues of social justice (Peabody, 2013).

Participatory video (PV) has been described by Lunch and Lunch (2006) as:

> a set of techniques to involve a group or community in shaping and creating their own film. The idea behind this is that making a video is easy and accessible, and is a great way of bringing people together to explore issues, voice concerns or simply to be creative and tell stories. (p. 10)

PV as increasingly carried out through cellphones and other devices (Mitchell, Delange, & Moletsane, 2017) makes available for children and youth opportunities to spontaneously record what they see through their own eyes, providing a child-based understanding of knowledge that is focused in their neighborhood (Pink, 2001; Sandercock & Attili, 2010). PV minimizes reliance on literacy skills and allows communicating a message without a reliance on writing or reading and as a result, becomes an "equalizing" tool (Okahashi, 2000). The process of videotaping, editing, and screening can be educational and therapeutic giving way to personal growth (Sandercock & Attili, 2010). Additionally, the use of PV promotes participation and encourages the right to have a voice and therefore "has long term implications for participatory citizenship" (Pascal & Bertram, 2009, p. 249).

Children and youth have increasingly available multimedia tools and a wide array of social network platforms which provide them opportunities to share their stories by using their own voices through digital storytelling. Digital storytelling is a "workshop-based process by which "ordinary people" create their own short autobiographical films that can be streamed on the Web or broadcast on television' (Burgess, 2006, p. 207). Children's stories are expressed by using a combination of methods such as images, drawings, voice and videos to develop a short (3- to 5-minute) digital story to share with others. These child-led productions, by using multiple modalities, "can be a transformative experience due to its potential for their meaningful engagement with their topic and engagement in deeper learning, critical reflection, meaning-making, self-expression, and effective communication" (D'Amico et al., 2016, p. 537).

Other tools that are "low tech" such as drawing, painting, and mapmaking have been used with children and youth affected by global adversity to better understand their experiences and the way that they see and understand the world. As D'Amico et al. (2016) argue, these visual tools create an environment where the children and youth may be more at ease and therefore, feel more capable to express themselves freely, and do not feel as much of a risk of giving a "wrong" answer as they may experience in interviews. Visual representations, in combination with other approaches that additionally elicit a narrative/story, make it possible to help children and youth convey aspects of their lived experiences in myriad ways (Leitch, 2008). Clinically, these tools have been used to better understand children's knowledge and experiences and at times are used as adjunct to diagnostic assessment tools.

Finally, various researchers and practitioners have made use of live performance. In Image theatre, participants use their bodies as a visual language to convey their lived experience (Boal, 1979; Linds & Vettraino, 2008). For example, one technique involves an individual telling a story as others silently use their bodies to visually represent a significant moment in the story. As D'Amico et al. (2016) note, the image or "tableau" can then be handled in different ways for example, of fast forwarding to the future or rewinding to events in the past, enabling a "manipulation" of time and space. Boal (as cited in Jackson, 1992) adds that images created through participation "offer a screen onto which a group can project a variety of ideas and interpretations" (p. 174), inviting the individual and the collective to problem solve. In groups with varying levels of verbal or linguistic ability, Image theatre minimizes the difference and becomes a common visual language. The "image-making provided the youth with a way to both create distance from and illuminate the ethos of violence in which they are steeped" (Kuftinec, 2011, p. 114). This allows for enabling an exploration of possibilities for change from, and through, the embodied image and "activating the youths' imagination of a world without violence and how to get there" (D'Amico et al., 2016, p. 536).

Toward a framework for the use of the arts in family practices in social work education

In this section we draw together what we see as a promising convergence of two bodies of literature, previous work on the arts in social work practice and previous work on the arts in work with war affected youth and their families. By bringing them together in one section, we propose an arts framework in family practice in social work education. (see Figure 1)

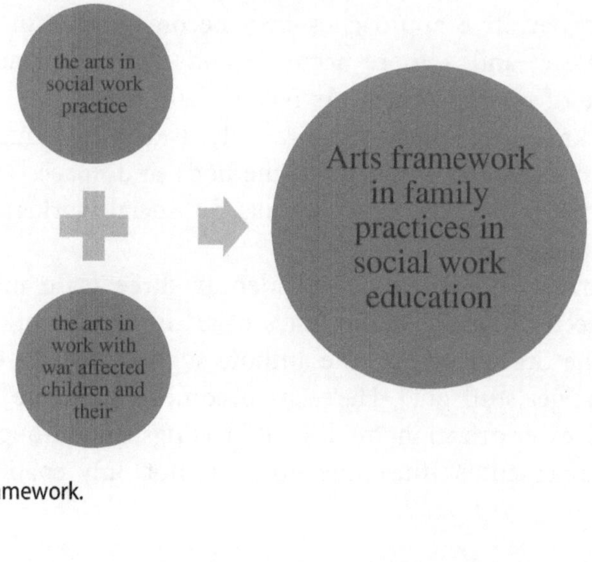

Figure 1. Arts framework.

Social work and the arts: history and context

Social work as a discipline and a profession has historically engaged with art. As far back as the settlement house movement in the late 1800s, social work has incorporated the arts in community action by forming partnerships with artists in addressing social issues and human challenges (Moxley & Feen, 2016). Yet the 20th century saw a powerful movement away from artistic endeavors, toward scientific methods, standardized efficacy, and ethical reliability (Cohen Konrad, 2017). Mary Richmond's pioneering of the scientific method in social casework and the emphasis on social diagnosis dominated the profession for decades (Richmond, 1917; 1922). This approach retained preeminence until the 1960s when the reemergence of protest movements reawakened social work's desire to recapture its identity as an empowerment movement (Cohen Konrad, 2017).

Yet in the contemporary context, social workers are increasingly challenged to work within the realities of burgeoning caseloads, managerial checklists, intense bureaucracies, and reduced quality time with clients. Many scholars and practitioners have warned against the dangers of this neoliberalistic approach seeping into all realms of social work, rendering it a mechanical, heavily regulated, and assembly-line series of practices. Craig (2007) argues that social workers have become experts in using a "scientific" and "neutral" voice. And yet, science alone may be inadequate for conveying the nuances and complexities of the human situation. Many scholars and practitioners assert that the focus on managerialism and mechanistic practices have resulted in the repression of social work as a creative endeavor (Huss & Sela-Amit, 2018) and to a "debasement of [the] craft" (Fabricant, 1985, p. 393). In a context of increasing practitioner stress, and ethical challenges, van Wormer (2002) has called for the protection of the "social work imagination" (p. 21), and there continues to be debates and conflicts as to what social work "is" and "is not" (Nissen, 2017). In this sense, art, storytelling and narrative approaches may become forms of resistance to the scientific voice, and a more accurate and nuanced window into the lived experience of social workers. As Nissen (2017) asserts, "we must deny the belief that knowledge and truth are only available through linear and increasingly neoliberalized social work methods and spaces" (p. 6). Given these realities, there have been recent calls for social workers to return to their artistic roots.

Sinding, Warren, and Paton (2014) identify three main metaphors that describe the effectiveness and importance of art in social work practice and education. In the first metaphor, the authors suggest that art enables social work clients to "get stuff out." Here, art becomes an avenue to enable the expression and exteriorization of difficult feelings and thoughts, allowing troubles to be released. At the same time, art not only enables feelings to "get out," but also that art "gets in"—actively able to reach meaningful and emotional depths not readily accessible otherwise. In the second metaphor, Sinding et al. (2014) argue that art helps clients to "inhabit other worlds." Moving well beyond the cognitive, art is sensory, activates emotion, and enables clients to safely and imaginatively enter or come closer to "walking in another's shoes" and others' lived experiences. Finally, they suggest that art "breaks habits" of seeing and knowing. Art interrupts patterns of seeing and knowing defined by stereotypes and prejudice—turning our attention to these habits and creating possibilities for new ways of knowing and relating.

Art may be increasingly valuable on macro-, mezzo-, and microlevels. Grassau (2009) suggested that the arts have particular value in uncovering "relational and structural aspects of oppression" (p. 249) that is so critical to social values and practice in community social work. The use of the arts in group work can enable participants to create highly supportive intentional communities, which can strengthen group cohesion, develop group identity, and foster social action among people who experience stigma, marginalization, and/or exclusion (Green & Denov, 2018). Through collaborative and interdisciplinary projects and coalitions, social workers and artists may partner in a broad forms of social action to bring about change at the micro-, mezzo-, and macrolevels (Moxley & Feen, 2016). On a more micro, practitioner level, art also has the capacity to increase reflexivity. Reflexive practice adopts a critical stance, compelling the practitioner to reflect on the ways in which power relations and social location embody and shape our interactions with clients. Moreover, because the arts are primarily a communicative medium, they can enhance communication between social workers and clients (Huss & Sela-Amit, 2018). Moxley and Feen (2016) suggest that the arts can strengthen praxis advancing the integration of theory and practice when "those involved in social work practice move from artful conceptions or images of social issues to the design and testing of helping strategies" (p. 1691).

The neurobiological basis of art must also be considered. The arts are said to induce prompt perceptual processing, information gathering, and metabolic arousal that mobilize the organism for coping reactions (Huss & Sela-Amit, 2018). On a deep neurological level, art is a personal interpretation of a social context that connects to problem solving and resilience (Sarid & Huss, 2010).

Within the realm of research, using art can provide powerful and highly accessible mechanisms for research dissemination (McNiff, 2008). More easily distributed, accessed, and consumed than traditional academic publications, these mediums can have a widespread, immediate, and powerful impact (Evans & Foster, 2009). Also, methods that put production in the hands of service users can project a credibility and authenticity that more polished works of art cannot achieve, provoking social action and potential social transformation (McNiff, 2008).

Calls for the use of the arts in social work curriculum

Within an increasingly austere, market-driven, and individually focused social context, the way that social work education has prepared students has altered considerably, and it has been argued that changes to the educational process and mission of universities have undermined the creativity and autonomy of the academy (Leonard, Hafford-Letchfield, & Couchman, 2018). The search for novel and innovative approaches has led to an increasing interest in arts-based methods as a vehicle for social change, often borrowing methods from the arts to enrich social work pedagogy. Eadie and Lymbery (2007) suggested that social work education needs to balance the technical aspects of professional education with more creative aspects, which will enable future social workers to creatively and thoughtfully adapt to a changing world. Leonard et al. (2018) and Chambon (2009) assert that introducing the arts in social work pedagogy offers opportunities for students and practitioners to foster different learning styles and varied ways of knowing and understanding in varied contexts. Schubert and Gray (2015) note that different interpretations through the arts could help enhance diagnostic, analytic, and action capabilities of social work in collaboration with service users in new ways of practicing. Huss and Sela-Amit (2018) argue that the arts can provide a space for social work students, as well as for service users, to excavate their own emotions and understanding of their work. This, in turn, can disrupt automatic thinking in a critically reflective space—a key goal of social work education and supervision. Kirkendall and Krishen (2014) have similarly asserted the need for creativity in the classroom, inviting students to "define creativity, suggest methods to infuse it in the classroom, and apply it as practitioners" (p. 341). However, when exploring students interest in art and creativing, Kirkendall and Krishen found that though students in the classroom were committed and willing to engage creatively, time restrictions, traditional classroom arrangements, and prescribed classroom assignments and formats inhibited more creative forms of learning and engagement.

Children, families, war, and the arts

Arts-based approaches to working with war-affected children and families such as photography, video making, music, drama and visual arts, have been found to promote participant activism, engagement, and empowerment (Mitchell, 2011). Furthermore, arts-based approaches have psychological benefits, as they provide a means for communicating with the nonverbal mind, and a way to safely access traumatic memory, making them an ideal vehicle for helping with traumatic recovery (Coleman & Macintosh, 2015; Gantt & Tinnin, 2009). Hobfoll et al. (2007) put together a panel of experts to identify the essential elements of immediate and midterm interventions when there has been mass trauma. They describe five guiding principles to include "a sense of safety, calming, a sense of self-and-community efficacy, connectedness, and hope" (p. 284). Betancourt, Meyers-Ohki, Charrow, and Tol (2013) undertook a systematic review of intervention with children affected by war. Betancourt et al. (2013) found the following strong evidence:

> secure and consistent caregiving relationships are critical in order for children to weather the extreme stressors of war and conflict. As a result, a number of psychosocial interventions are oriented toward the family, with the aim of strengthening parent-child relationships and connection. (p. 80)

In this section we draw attention to two arts-based interventions with war-affected children that seem particularly relevant to families and family practice. We do not offer this as an exhaustive systematic review, but rather as an "aperçu" on examples of different arts-based practices in working with war-affected children, youth, families, and communities in multiple contexts, either in areas affected by war or on refugees.

Arts-based intervention with refugee children in a Canadian context

Yohani (2008) conducted an arts based project in a Canadian city where arts-based tools were used as a tool of data gathering and a set of activities to enhance and develop hope among refugee children and their families. The study focused on fourteen refugee children from ages 8 to 18 who had spent time in a third-world country before coming to Canada. Building on key ideas on the nature of hope, the project used photographs, a hope quilt, and the development of stories where children shared their work with others and, through this, enabled adults to carry out child-focused discussions. Hope was explored through collage, drawing, painting, and photography as "these arts-based approaches were particularly relevant since hope is associated with creative processes (Lynch, 1965) and these activities are considered developmentally appropriate for eliciting information in children of this age" (van Manen, 1994, p. 315). Children's photographs depicted images taken in their homes, schools, classrooms, after-school care programs, parks, and neighborhoods. A "hope quilt" depicted the stories of the children providing them with another medium for the children to "explore their experiences of hope and allowed children to move beyond their current contexts and reflect on past experiences and future goals" (Yohani, 2008 p. 312). The children then shared the hope quilt in a small exhibit.

Yohani (2008) noted that at the time of publication of her article, little had been documented on how refugee children adapt to their new countries. She underlined that "a better understanding of children's successes and failures holds the potential to contribute to both theory and practice on this subject" (p. 310). Using Bronfenbrenner's (1979) bioecological theory of human development, she developed appropriate arts-based activities to help the researcher understand the realities of children's lives in the new country. In bioecological theory, the term *ecology* refers to the range of situations people are involved in, from their roles, the challenges they encounter and what happens thus "a key component of this theory is its attention to person, process, context, and time" (Yohani, 2008, p. 311). Interactions between people and their environment are strongly influenced by individual or personal factors such as emotions, be it anger or happiness. Hope may be one of these emotions. It is often embedded in personal experiences and life contexts; it is nurtured in reciprocal relationships and involves action and personal appraisal of actions. Yohani pointed out "these aspects of hope bear relevance in work with at-risk refugee children, specifically with interventions aimed at engendering hope in children by strengthening connections to themselves and to people within their milieu" (p. 311).

The researcher also involved adult program staff and parents to look at what emerged for the children in terms of hope. Beginning with discussions of the dark side of hope, parents transformed their focus to hope itself. Interestingly, once findings regarding children's perceptions were shared, parents and cultural brokers began to change their discussion to reflect more hopeful language:

> One parent expressed surprise at viewing her daughter's work and talked about working hard to make her daughter feel proud of who she was. She had watched her child struggle at school and now that she was starting to do well, it pleased the mother to see that her daughter had begun to envision herself in the future. (p. 312)

The ecological framework, which included adult perspectives, helped contextualize hope in children's adjustment in the new country and demonstrated that hope radiated from children to adults and vice versa.

The arts in performance: healing intergenerational trauma as a result of war and its aftermath

The arts in performance can be a helpful approach to dealing with war and its aftermath. Erzar (2017) worked with three generations of Slovenians in an art therapy project, which was organized by a civil society organization to commemorate the 70th anniversary of the Second World War and postwar violence in that country. "The purpose of the event was to help former wartime children (now adults), victims of war and postwar violence, and their families to begin the process of mourning" (Erzar, 2017, p. 41). The researcher/therapists felt there were intergenerational effects of trauma that prevented families from recovering from the emotions and dysfunction that has resulted. To address these intergenerational aspects, the event involved the first generation who experienced the original trauma as those who invited participants, the second generation organized the event, and the third generation (i.e., the grandchildren of the first generation) as performers. The researchers found that each generation were touched in unique ways.

The researchers drew on the work of Kahane-Nissenbaum (2011) who studied the effects and consequences of trauma on three generations of the same family. For the first generation, halting or ending the trauma was a priority as "the major achievement of the war generation is thus to allow themselves to feel the fear and accept mistrust as part of their lives, while letting their children live without fear and mistrust" (p. 43). The task for the second generation was less about securing survival, but more about dealing with the trauma emotionally:

> If they are helped with the understanding that their parents survived the trauma (which is why they rarely enjoyed a relaxed childhood), the second-generation children are able to redirect attention from the past to their present relationships and the emotional side of life. (p. 43)

For the third generation, "their task is to know themselves better, turn to the world, and dream about the creation of a new one" (p. 43). Importantly for arts-based research and therapy, this third generation has a feeling for creativity and creating new worlds. However, if their parents could not redirect their fears to the potential of their children, their potential would not be fulfilled, "Despite the fact that they face no external threats and have no existential problems, these young people lack creativity and curiosity and have great difficulty getting in touch with the emotional side of their lives" (p. 43).

The Flowers of Compassion project aimed to open a space for mourning and reconciliation mainly through sensitive and emotionally accomplished artistic performances (music, theater, and exhibitions). Erzar (2017) reported on one part of this event, a concert held in 2015 that was devoted to the three generations, especially those who had not found where their grandparents who had been killed in the postwar reprisals were buried. The concert was conceived as a place to process the effects associated with injustice and resentment. The choice of music created the atmosphere, beginning with the *Fauré Requiem*, which introduced themes of loss and grief, followed by the premiere of a Slovenian war requiem, which offered hope for the future. The concert also included Slovenian poetry and paintings by a Slovenian artist who had lost three adolescent brothers during the war. This artist had survived the war's emotional effects as a child by creating emotional safety by drawing and painting.

Resolving the intergenerational transmission of fear, distrust, and violence requires a deep and lengthy process that starts with the reduction of anger and resentment and continues with the acknowledgment and empathic acceptance of pain (Shoshan, 1989). Artistic experience can add to this process by dismantling defensive reactions and revealing the layers of soft emotions beneath anger and resentment. Feelings of sadness, relief, and vulnerability are opened up through music, theater, film, literature, and painting, allowing individuals to get in touch with their inner pain and experience compassion (Erzar, 2017, p. 44). The responses of each generation indicated an effect. For the first generation, they "mentioned two fundamental emotions: sadness, expressed with tears and crying, and respect or dignity" (p. 46). For the second generation, they went "deeper into feelings of shame and abandonment … saying, their 'childhood feelings related to the injustice suffered by his parents were not unique and were perfectly understandable'" (p. 46). For the third generation, there was:

> cognitive acknowledgement of the war and postwar traumas, and emotional confusion regarding what is expected of responsible grandchildren. Young people see the stories of their grandparents as linked to a distant past they would like to see incorporated into the reality of their present lives. (p. 47)

By inviting three generations of one family, the artistic event showed what was possible to heal intergenerational trauma as a result of war.

To return to our "beginning at the beginning" question posed in the Introduction, how can the work described in the previous section inform social work practice with war-affected children and their families and what are the implications for social work education? Mazza (2009) wrote an introduction to an issue of the *Journal of Family Social Work* that called for the use of creative and artistic work in family social work. He pointed out that it is a matter of ethics for the family social worker to be able to recognize a family's unique history, strengths, and context (Mazza, 2009). Grassau (2009) also has called for increased use of visual images in social work given that some experiences are "below words" (p. 253). Indeed, given the tragedy of war and genocide, words and narrative alone often cannot adequately capture the realities and complexity of conflict-related experiences. As such, researchers focused on the fallout of war and genocide are increasingly turning to the arts to enable multiple forms of participant expression, as well as for the therapeutic, restorative and empowering qualities of arts-based techniques (Denov, Doucet, & Kamara, 2012). And yet, though art has been deemed a powerful tool when working with war-affected children and youth, its use with families has been explored far less. This is clearly an area of importance that begs further attention and research. As Mazza (2009) observed:

> Healing, growth, and awareness can be developed through the appreciation or creation of artistic works. Although the arts in family practice are particularly well suited for narrative therapy, it should be noted that poetic elements (e.g., use of metaphor, reframing, behavioral enactment, sculpting, music, genograms, scripts,

and family drawings) have been incorporated in all theoretical models of family therapy. (p. x)

In the next section, then, we offer a set of pedagogical features of arts-based work in professional practice that align well with well-established approaches to working with war-affected children and their families.

Social work practice with war-affected children and their families: some pedagogical features of arts-based approaches

An arts-based pedagogical orientation links well to creative and participatory strategies that have been tested out in a variety of professional contexts where empathy and social change are key (Mitchell, Weber, & Pithouse, 2009; Pithouse, Mitchell, & Moletsane, 2009). Although these (see Figure 2) are pedagogical features that could cut across an entire curriculum or program in a School of Social Work or a Faculty of Education, they could also be features that are more apparent in one or several courses or practicum experiences focusing on family practice.

Pedagogical features of arts-based practices

Reflexivity

Our framework begins with reflexivity. As is highlighted across a variety of fields of professional practice, instilling the importance of reflective processes in students is essential to securing ethical and safe social work practice in future work with vulnerable populations over the course of a career (Samson, 2015). To take one example, research suggests that interacting with authority figures after lengthy immigration processes is often a source of trauma for resettled refugees (George, 2012). New social work students may not have

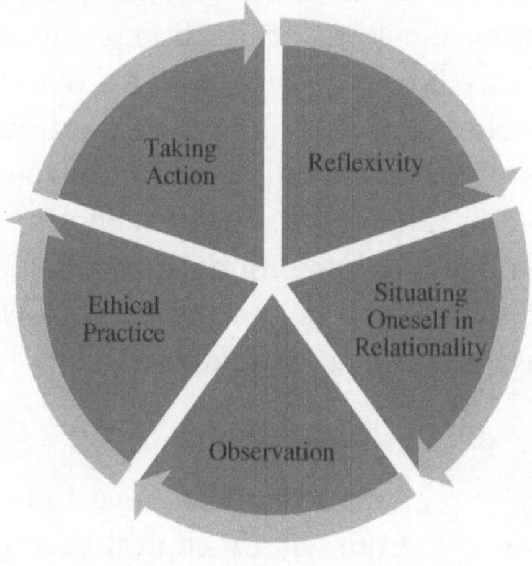

Figure 2. Pedagogical features.

developed the reflexivity to realize that they themselves represent a profession that can be experienced as an instrument of social control by those they serve and not the practice of promoting social justice as the student coming into social work may believe. The many films portraying professionals such as teachers coming into community practice with, for example, inner-city youth as we see in *Dangerous Minds* (Simpson, Bruckheimer, & Smith, 1995) highlight this dichotomy with a particular astuteness, and allowing new professionals to "see ourselves as others see us" and to consider how they themselves will navigate the formation of their professional identity (Clarke, Lovelock, & McNay, 2016). The "perspective-taking" process in holistic humanities educational activities closely resembles the linkages between individuals, family, community, environmental, and multicultural influences (Moxley & Feen, 2016). By breaking habitual ways of seeing and knowing there is more cognitive and affective space to see and know in more deeply perceptive ways and serve clients more effectively.

Situating oneself in relationality

Critical reflection is linking to situating oneself, an activity that can also be enhanced by the arts (Eisner, 2008; Giles & Pockett, 2013). Arts-based explorations can help to illuminate a student's relationship to privilege, race, oppression, and their own as well as others' lived experiences of vulnerability within social work practice (Leonard et al., 2018; Trevelyan, Crath, & Chambon, 2012). The simple act of expanding client histories with relevant visual arts, literature, and cinema among other art forms could powerfully transform common educational case studies into instruments that reveal the multilayered nature of client experience within its sociocultural context. Placing the arts at the center of conversations about war, race, class, social inequality, oppression, and injustice creates a learning environment that is provocative in relation to difficult pedagogical material, and at the same time remaining engaging, stimulating, and enjoyable. Exploring narratives from the clients' perspectives, multicultural literature, and other forms of cultural production precipitated by social realities offers a reasonable balance between these two vital objectives. As an example, Greek social work schools have successfully created art-based modules to assist students' deeper understanding and ability to ethically assess various facets of the European refugee crisis (Papouli, 2017). Such efforts have been mirrored in the United States by photography exhibitions showcasing the dignity and everydayness of the lives of asylum seekers as a way to visually deconstruct popular racist discourses by engaging empathy (Sinding et al., 2014).

Observation

Arts-based methodologies produce a richly emotive and embodied data set for practitioners to draw insight from, clarify clinical decision-making processes, and ultimately better serve their clients. One technique noted for its broad appeal and accessibility is Photovoice (Wang & Burris, 1997 ; Mitchell, 2011). This method allows for opportunity to engage the aesthetic impulse without impeding barriers of literacy, self-assessed artistic skill, language, or culture barring the way. Photovoice has been found to be an excellent method in assisting intercultural social work classrooms in exploring their personal and professional values in a more engaging, experiential and reflexive way than prevailing teaching methods (Bromfield & Capous-Desyllas, 2017). There is a direct translation of its utility in the classroom to its utility in community social work. In one such instance a Photovoice project at the undergraduate social work level became a community Photovoice project due to its broad accessibility and appeal (Bonnycastle & Bonnycastle, 2015). The photographs and photographers' explanation of them can help elucidate complex interactions between individuals' physical health, psychology, family systems, the community, sociocultural context, and political economy's influence with depth and intimacy (George, 2012; Murray, Lampinen, & Kelley-Soderholm, 2006).

Ethical practice

Arguably ethics and ethical practice in relation to war-affected children are most directly studied and appreciated through participatory arts-based methods that involve the production of artistic creations such as photos, cellphilms, and drawings. As highlighted by Akesson et al. (2014), issues such as voice, ownership, and interpretation become particularly critical. However, learning how and why such issues are so significant could take a "starting with ourselves" approach (van Manen, 1994) in social work education through learning by doing. How, for example, do we feel when working in group and one's individual voice and even one's individual contributions take second place to the group voice? How might we understand the tensions between individual response and collectivity?

Taking action

Finally, we consider the ways that training in innovative arts-based methodologies in the social work classroom can contribute to a new generation of arts-based practitioners engaged in taking action. Using a "learning by doing approach" students can delve into the process of working with the arts within their learning communities to focus on discovery and becoming as opposed to outcome and expectation (Crociani-Windland, 2017). The case of social work students producing anti-oppression 'zines is one such compelling example (Desyllas & Sinclair, 2014).

Conclusion

"… is it perhaps vital now more than ever to use the arts to disrupt status quo in social work education, research, and practice?"

(Cohen Konrad, 2017, p. 4).

Clearly, as in all realms, art cannot be considered a panacea in an increasingly complex and changing global context. Huss and Sela-Amit (2018, p. 1) introduce an important question, can social workers really afford to include the arts in a context of limited client-time, and when these clients are facing real-world problems, such as accessing basic needs such as food and shelter? Moreover, the power relations that exist between social workers and clients do not disappear or transcend methodological challenges and problems. As in all social work interventions, there is a danger that art can become a tool of oppression within power-infused interactions between social workers and clients. In addition, social work's use of art occurs within a specific cultural and sociogeographic context. All creations need to be defined by its creator and should not be a fine art disconnected from its creator. In this sense, when embracing the arts, social work students and practitioners needs to be aware of social work`s western roots, paradigms, and ways of seeing, ensuring the unique cultural, social and contextual meaning and significance of the art is expressed by clients and not social work students and practitioners. The suitability of art as a method and interaction with clients and families must be carefully assessed, particularly in relation to context and culture. At the same time, and in closing, our answer to Cohen Konrad's (2017) question posed above remains overwhelmingly in the affirmative. As the burgeoning body of work with war affected youth and their families highlights, it is critical "now more than ever" to find methods and tools in professional practice that recognize the healing potential and their potential to deepen an understanding of the issues. A good place to begin is at the beginning.

Disclosure statement

No potential conflict of interest was reported by the authors.

Funding

This work was supported by the Fonds de Recherche du Québec-Société et Culture (2017-SE-196298).

ORCID

Claudia Mitchell http://orcid.org/0000-0002-9790-2486

References

Akesson, B., D'Amico, M., Denov, M., Khan, F., Linds, W., & Mitchell, C. A. (2014). 'Stepping back 'as researchers: Addressing ethics in arts-based approaches to working with war-affected children in school and community settings. *Educational Research for Social Change*, *3*(1), 75–89. doi:10.1080/17441692.2016.1165719

Betancourt, T. S., Meyers-Ohki, M. S. E., Charrow, M. A. P., & Tol, W. A. (2013). Interventions for children affected by war: An ecological perspective on psychosocial support and mental health care. *Harvard Review of Psychiatry*, *21*(2), 70–91. doi:10.1097/HRP.0b013e318283bf8f

Boal, A. (1979). *Theatre of the oppressed*. Trans. Charles A. and Maria-Odilia Leal McBride. L. London, UK: Pluto Press.

Bonnycastle, M. M., & Bonnycastle, C. R. (2015). Photographs generate knowledge: Reflections on experiential learning in/outside the social work classroom. *Journal of Teaching in Social Work*, *35*(3), 233–250. doi:10.1080/08841233.2015.1027031

Bromfield, N. F., & Capous-Desyllas, M. (2017). Photovoice as a pedagogical tool: Exploring personal and professional values with female Muslim social work students in an intercultural classroom setting. *Journal of Teaching in Social Work*, *37*(5), 493–512. doi:10.1080/08841233.2017.1380744

Bronfenbrenner, U. (1979). *The ecology of human development*. Cambridge, MA: Harvard University Press.

Burgess, J. (2006). Hearing ordinary voices: Cultural studies, vernacular creativity and digital storytelling. *Continuum: Journal of Media & Cultural Studies*, *20*(2), 201–214. doi:10.1080/10304310600641737

Chambon, A. (2009). What can art do for social work? *Canadian Social Work Review*, *26*(2), 217–231. Retrieved from http://www.jstor.org/stable/41669914

Clarke, J., Lovelock, R., & McNay, M. (2016). Liberal arts and the development of emotional intelligence in social work education. *The British Journal of Social Work*, *46*(3), 635–651. doi:10.1093/bjsw/bcu139

Cohen Konrad, S. (2017). Art in social work: Equivocation, evidence and ethical quandaries. *Research on Social Work Practice*, 1–5. doi:10.1177/1049731517735898

Coleman, K., & Macintosh, H. B. (2015). Art and evidence: Balancing the discussion on arts-and evidence-based practices with traumatized children. *Journal of Child & Adolescent Trauma*, *8*(1), 21–31. doi:10.1007/s40653-015-0036-1

Craig, R. (2007). A day in the life of a hospital social worker. *Qualitative Social Work*, *6*(4), 431–446. doi:10.1177/1473325007083355

Crociani-Windland, L. (2017). Deleuze, art and social work. *Journal of Social Work Practice*, *31*(2), 251–262. doi:10.1080/02650533.2017.1305341

D'Amico, M., Denov, M., Khan, F., Linds, W., & Akesson, B. (2016). Research as intervention? Exploring the health and well-being of children and youth facing global adversity through participatory visual methods. *Global Public Health*, *11*(5–6), 528–545. doi:10.1080/17441692.2016.1165719

Denov, M., Doucet, D., & Kamara, A. (2012). Engaging war-affected youth through photography: Photovoice with child soldiers in Sierra Leone. *Intervention*, *10*(2), 117–133. doi:10.1097/WTF.0b013e328355ed82

Desyllas, M. C., & Sinclair, A. (2014). Zine-making as a pedagogical tool for transformative learning in social work education. *Social Work Education*, *33*(3), 296–316. doi:10.1080/02615479.2013.805194

Eadie, T., & Lymbery, M. (2007). Promoting creative practice through social work education. *Social Work Education*, *26*(7), 670–683. doi:10.1080/02615470601129842

Eisner, E. (2008). Art and knowledge. In J. G. Knowles & A. L. Cole (Eds.), *Handbook of the arts in qualitative research: Perspectives, methodologies, examples, and issues* (pp. 3–12). Thousand Oaks, CA: Sage.

Erzar, K. (2017). The Flowers of Compassion: A trauma-informed artistic event involving three generations of Slovenians (Les fleurs de la compassion: Un événement artistique qui tient compte du traumatisme de trois générations de slovéniens et les implique). *Canadian Art Therapy Association Journal, 30*(1), 41–49. doi:10.1080/08322473.2017.1303862

Evans, M., & Foster, S. (2009). Representation in participatory video: Some considerations from research with Métis in British Columbia. *Journal of Canadian Studies, 43*(1), 87–108. doi:10.3138/jcs.43.1.87

Fabricant, M. (1985). The industrialization of social work practice. *Social Work, 30*(5), 389–395. doi:10.1093/sw/30.5.389

Foster, V. (2012). What if? The use of poetry to promote social justice. *Social Work Education, 31*(6), 742–755. doi:10.1080/02615479.2012.695936

Gangi, J. M., & Barowsky, E. (2009). Listening to children's voices: Literature and the arts as means of responding to the effects of war, terrorism, and disaster. *Childhood Education, 85* (6), 357–363. doi:10.1080/00094056.2009.10521401

Gantt, L., & Tinnin, L. (2009). Support for a neurobiological view of trauma with implications for art therapy. *The Arts in Psychotherapy, 36*(3), 148–153. doi:10.1016/j.aip.2008.12.005

George, M. (2012). Migration traumatic experiences and refugee distress: Implications for social work practice. *Clinical Social Work Journal, 40*(4), 429–437. doi:10.1007/s10615-012-0397-y

Giles, R., & Pockett, R. (2013). Critical reflection in social work education. In J. Fook & F. Gardner (Eds.), *Critical reflection in context* (pp. 208–218). London, UK: Routledge.

Grassau, P. (2009). Resilience and 'turning it out': How the arts engage with relational and structural aspects of oppression. *Canadian Social Work Review, 26*(2), 249–265. Retrieved from http://www.jstor.org/stable/41669916

Green, A., & Denov, M. (2018). Mask-making and drawing as method: An arts-based approach to data collection with war-affected children. *International Journal of Qualitative Research.* In Press.

Harris, D. A. (2007). Pathways to embodied empathy and reconciliation after atrocity: Former boy soldiers in a dance/movement therapy group in Sierra Leone. *Intervention, 5*(3), 203–231. doi:10.1097/WTF.0b013e3282f211c8

Hobfoll, S. E., Watson, P., Bell, C. C., Bryant, R. A., Brymer, M. J., Friedman, & Ursana, R. J. (2007). Five essential elements of immediate and mid-term mass trauma intervention: Empirical evidence. *Psychiatry, 70*(4), 283–315. doi:10.1521/psyc.2007.70.4.283

Huss, E., & Sela-Amit, M. (2018). Art in social work: Do we really need it? *Research on Social Work Practice*, 1–6. doi:10.1177/1049731517745995

Jackson, A. (1992). *Games for actors and non-actors.* (Translator's introduction to A. Boal). New York, NY: Taylor & Francis.

Jackson, K. (2015). Beyond talk- creative arts therapies in social work. *Social Work Today, 15* (3), 22. Retrieved from http://www.socialworktoday.com/archive/051815p22.shtml

Kahane-Nissenbaum, M. (2011). *Exploring intergenerational transmission of trauma in third generation of Holocaust survivors* (Doctoral Dissertation). University of Pennsylvania, Philadelphia, PA. Scholarly Commons.

Kirkendall, A., & Krishen, A. (2014). Encouraging creativity in the social work classroom: Insights from a qualitative exploration. *Social Work Education, 34*(3), 341–354. doi:10.1080/02615479.2014.986089

Kuftinec, S. (2011). Rehearsing for dramatic change in Kabul. In T. Emert & E. Friedland (Eds.), *Come closer: Critical perspectives on theatre of the oppressed* (pp. 109–116). New York, NY: Peter Lang.

Leitch, R. (2008). Creatively researching children's narratives through images and drawings. In P. Thomson (Ed.), *Doing visual research with children and young people* (pp. 37–58). London, UK: Taylor & Francis.

Leonard, K., Hafford-Letchfield, T., & Couchman, W. (2018). The impact of the arts in social work education: A systematic review. *Qualitative Social Work*, *17*(2), 286–304. doi:10.1177/1473325016662905

Linds, W., & Vettraino, E. (2008). Collective imagining: Collaborative story telling through image theater. *Forum Qualitative Sozialforschung/Forum: Qualitative Social Research*, *9*(2). Retrieved from http://nbn-resolving.de/urn:nbn:de:0114-fqs0802568

Lunch, N., & Lunch, C. (2006). *Insights into participatory video: A handbook for the field*. Oxford, UK: Insight.

Mazza, N. (2009). The arts and family social work: A call for advancing practice, research, and education. *Journal of Family Social Work*, *12*(1), 3–8. doi:10.1080/10522150802383084

McNiff, S. (2008). Arts-based research. In J. G. Knowles & A. L. Cole (Eds.), *Handbook of the arts in qualitative research: Perspectives, methodologies, examples, and issues* (pp. 29–40). London, UK: Sage.

Mitchell, C. (2011). *Doing Visual Research*. London, UK: Sage.

Mitchell, C., Delange, N., & Moletsane, R. (2017). *Participatory visual methodologies: Social change, community and policy*. London, UK: Sage.

Mitchell, C., Weber, S., & Pithouse, K. (2009). Facing the public: Using photography for self-study and social action. In D. Tidwell, M. Heston, & L. Fitzgerald (Eds.), *Research methods for the self-study of practice* (pp. 119–134). New York, NY: Springer.

Moletsane, R., De Lange, N., Mitchell, C., Stuart, J., Buthelezi, T., & Taylor, M. (2007). Photo-voice as a tool for analysis and activism in response to HIV and AIDS stigmatisation in a rural KwaZulu-Natal school. *Journal of Child and Adolescent Mental Health*, *19*(1), 19–28. doi:10.2989/17280580709486632

Moxley, D., & Feen, H. (2016). Arts-inspired design in the development of helping interventions in social work: Implications for the integration of research and practice. *British Journal of Social Work*, *46*(6), 1690–1707. doi:10.1093/bjsw/bcv087

Murray, C. E., Lampinen, A., & Kelley-Soderholm, E. L. (2006). Teaching family systems theory through service-learning. *Counselor Education and Supervision*, *46*(1), 44–58. doi:10.1002/j.1556-6978.2006.tb00011.x

Nissen, L. B. (2017). Art and social work: History and collaborative possibilities for interdisciplinary synergy. *Research on Social Work Practice*, 1–10. doi:10.1177/1049731517733804

Okahashi, P. (2000). The potential of participatory video. *Rehabilitation Review*, *11*(1), 1–4. Retrieved from wwwmcc.murdoch.edu.au/ReadingRoom/3.2/Tomaselli.html

Osofsky, J. D., & Osofsky, H. J. (2018). Challenges in building child and family resilience after disasters. *Journal of Family Social Work*, 1–14. doi:10.1080/10522158.2018.1427644

Papouli, E. (2017). The role of arts in raising ethical awareness and knowledge of the European refugee crisis among social work students. An example from the classroom. *Social Work Education*, *36*(7), 775–793. doi:10.1080/02615479.2017.1353074

Pascal, C., & Bertram, T. (2009). Listening to young citizens: The struggle to make real a participatory paradigm in research with young children. *European Early Childhood Education Research Journal*, *17*(2), 249–262. doi:10.1080/13502930902951486

Peabody, C. G. (2013). Using photovoice as a tool to engage social work students in social justice. *Journal of Teaching in Social Work*, *33*(3), 251–265. doi:10.1080/08841233.2013.795922

Pink, S. (2001). *Doing visual ethnography*. London, UK: Sage.

Pithouse, K., Mitchell, C., & Moletsane, R. (Eds.). (2009). *Making connections: Self-study and social action* (Vol. 357). New York, NY: Peter Lang.

Richmond, M. E. (1917). *Social diagnosis*. New York, NY: Russell Sage Foundation.

Richmond, M. E. (1922). *What is social case work? an introductory description*. New York, NY: Russell Sage Foundation.

Samson, P. L. (2015). Practice wisdom: The art and science of social work. *Journal of Social Work Practice, 29*(2), 119–131. doi:10.1080/02650533.2014.922058

Sandercock, L., & Attili, G. (2010). Digital ethnography as planning praxis: An experiment with film as social research, community engagement and policy dialogue. *Planning Theory and Practice, 11*(1), 23–45. doi:10.1080/14649350903538012

Sarid, O., & Huss, E. (2010). Trauma and acute stress disorder: A comparison between cognitive behavioural intervention and art therapy. *The Arts in Psychotherapy, 37*(1), 8–12. doi:10.1016/j.aip.2009.11.004

Schubert, L., & Gray, M. (2015). The death of emancipatory social work as art and birth of socially engaged art practice. *British Journal of Social Work, 45*(4), 1349–1356. doi:10.1093/bjsw/bcv020

Shoshan, T. (1989). Mourning and longing from generation to generation. *American Journal of Psychotherapy, 43*(2), 193–207. doi:10.1176/appi.psychotherapy.1989.43.2.193

Simpson, D, & Bruckheimer, J. (1995). *Dangerous minds* [Motion picture]. USA: Hollywood Pictures.

Sinding, C., Warren, R., & Paton, C. (2014). Social work and the arts: Images at the intersection. *Qualitative Social Work, 13*(2), 187–202. doi:10.1177/1473325012464384

Trevelyan, C., Crath, R., & Chambon, A. (2012). Promoting critical reflexivity through arts-based media: A case study. *British Journal of Social Work, 44*(1), 7–26. doi:10.1093/bjsw/bcs090

van Manen, M. (1994). *Researching lived experience: Human Science for an Action Sensitive Pedagogy*. London, Ontario: The Althouse Press.

van Wormer, K. (2002). Our social work imagination. *Journal of Teaching in Social Work, 22* (3–4), 21–37. doi:10.1300/J067v22n03_03

Wang, C., & Burris, M. (1997). Photovoice: Concept, methodology, and use for participatory needs assessment. *Health and Behaviour, 24*(3), 369–387. doi:10.1177/109019819702400309

Yohani, S. (2008). Creating an ecology of hope: Arts-based interventions with refugee children. *Child & Adolescent Social Work Journal, 25*(4), 309–323. doi:10.1007/s10560-008-0129-x

Culture, migration, and identity formation in adolescent refugees: a family perspective

Marjorie Aude Rabiau

ABSTRACT

Looking through a cultural lens at the family system level, expressions of distress in adolescent refugees are explored using the constructs of postmigration cultural identity formation and cultural idioms of distress. Asylum-seeking minors have heightened risk of developing mental health problems. Family is an important protective factor, and a sustained lack of parental figures further increases these young peoples' vulnerability to mental health problems. The family plays a significant role as an anchor to cultural identity. Case studies from a cultural consultation service in a clinical psychiatry department were used to illustrate two potential trajectories regarding identity formation and the impact on expressions of distress and family functioning. Case analysis also emphasized the clinical relevance of exploring meaning making and cultural idioms of distress in the face of trauma and loss at the individual and the family level. Clinical implications focus on a family and a cultural lens to emphasize the importance of contextualizing expressions of distress in adolescents who had to flee from war-affected areas.

Introduction

Adolescence is a time of increased vulnerability to external stressors and young refugees from war-torn countries are a particularly vulnerable group (Durà-Vilà, Klasen, Makatini, Rahimi, & Hodes, 2013; Hassan et al., 2015). Evans and Forte (2013) noted that one third of the global population of displaced people is thought to be between ages 10 and 24, with almost one half (47%) being younger than age 18. Asylum-seeking minors have heightened risk of developing mental health problems due to the stressors they have been exposed to in their home country (i.e., war, disruption to community life, witnessing deaths), in transit (i.e., separation from caregivers, illness), and upon arrival (i.e., uncertainty of refugee status, discrimination, low social support) (Derluyn & Broekaert, 2008; Fazel, Reed, Panter-Brick, & Stein, 2012). Depression and anxiety are very common among asylum-seeking adolescents and often occur alongside posttraumatic stress disorder (PTSD) (Ehntholt & Yule, 2006).

However, the applicability of Western mental health concepts and standardized measures to war-affected adolescents from other regions need to be reconsidered (Hassan et al., 2015) or at the very least understood in a larger context at the socioecological level (Denov, Fennig, Rabiau, & Shevell, in press). More specifically, expressions of distress and mental health symptoms need to be explored within the culture in which they are embedded. In this article, we define *culture* not as a static and unidimensional construct but rather as a dynamic process of meaning making (Hassan et al., 2015). Applying a strength-based culturally sensitive approach rather than focusing on an individual and deficiency-based model could deepen our understanding and improve services.

LeFrançois and Coppock (2014) introduced the very important point that to provide children and youth with a sense of agency we first need to deconstruct the social construction of childhood as incompetence and inferiority. They highlight the intersectionality of the notion of childhood with the notion mental health diagnosis as further denying children as "knowers," and therefore in need of receiving treatment from experts. This points to the importance for children and youth to be engaged in their own meaning making and to be engaged in decision making to feel a sense of agency. Rabaia, Saleh, and Giacaman (2014) further acknowledge the importance of this sense of agency in populations of children and youth who suffered the trauma of war. They point to the necessity of addressing macrosystemic issues and the root of their suffering rather than individualize the distress as pathology. We need to be cautious not to impose a model that excludes cultural and historical understanding. Moreover, Rabaia et al. (2014) stress the importance of empowerment and using a strength-based approach. They aptly remark that most research on war-affected children focus on prevalence levels of mental health symptoms and diagnoses while rarely asking the question of how the children and youth have managed to maintain their mental health amidst being exposed to horrendous violence.

Moving from macro- to microsystem, the family is an important microsystem within which culture and meaning making are transmitted and nurtured. McGregor, Melvin, and Newman (2015, 2016) describe the importance of family as a supportive factor for emotional and social support for resettled refugee youth. The presence of family members can transform adversity into a source of strength by aiding in the rebuilding of a meaningful universe. The family therefore appears to be an anchor for identity in exile (Rousseau, Mekki-Berrada, & Moreau, 2001). The construct of identity and identity formation will be elaborated on as a cohesive sense of identity has been shown to be an important protective factor for the adaptation and mental health of adolescent refugees (Fazel et al., 2012; Stevens & Walsh, 2016; Walsh et al., 2018).

Although asylum-seeking minors have a heightened risk of developing mental health problems, or at least experiencing distress not to fall into Western nomenclature, family is an important protective factor. A sustained lack of parental figure further increases young peoples' vulnerability (Hodes, Jagdev, Chandra, & Cunniff, 2008). For example, the authors of one study suggested that unaccompanied minors are five times more likely to have emotional difficulties than those who are accompanied by a caregiver (Derluyn, Broekaert, & Schuyten, 2008). Unaccompanied minors show higher levels of PTSD symptoms than accompanied minors and minors from nonrefugee populations (Huemer et al., 2009), as well as higher levels of anxiety (Derluyn & Broekaert, 2007). Family support and cohesion are related to better mental health for young refugees (Kovacev & Shute, 2004; Rousseau, Drapeau, & Platt, 2004), as is parental mental health (Betancourt, 2015; Hjern, Angel, & Jeppson, 1998). Family is an environmental buffer and source of resilience against traumas. Strengthening family ties and forging a supportive family milieu are important goals of intervention with youth and families. Jones (1998, 2014) ascertains that rebuilding the social and cultural milieu and the re-creation of social networks and communities is primordial.

When working with resettled refugees, contextualizing individuals' and families' experiences is key in fostering resilience and empowering the reconstruction of meaningful lives (Denov et al., in press). Denov et al. (in press) eloquently illustrate that stories matter. In this article, we discuss the importance of contextualizing expressions of distress in adolescents who had to flee from war-affected areas using a family and a cultural lens. Using case studies, we explore the constructs of postmigration identity formation and more specifically cultural identity formation. Finally, we discuss the clinical relevance of exploring meaning making and cultural idioms of distress in the face of trauma and loss at the individual and the family level.

The following quote from Jones (1998) encapsulates the essence of what we are setting up to explore in this article:

> The normal adolescent task of identity formation is more easily undertaken when the boundaries of family, peer group, community and country are stable, visible and defined. Choice as to what to identify with and with whom to make relationships, take place within a stable and clearly understood context. Not so for the adolescent refugee: how does one challenge the establishment when this has been swept away? What is one's own role when parents may be injured, dependent, missing or dead? How does one reconcile the conflicting claims or parents who may be demanding greater loyalty to ethnic identity, and the demands of the host country for rapid assimilation? And in a long war, how does one choose between a perceived duty to return and defend that country, or beginning again elsewhere? (p. 543)

How should social workers and mental health providers best support refugee youth from war-affected areas postmigration? Looking through a cultural lens at the family system level, many facets need to be reflected upon to obtain a holistic meaningful narrative. These facets include identity formation as a life-cycle transition, cultural identity formation, traumas and losses, family and social support, and meaning making and cultural idioms of distress. We develop each of these facets throughout the article.

Identity formation and individuation

Adolescence has been identified by Erik Erikson (1993) as a key period for exploring identity versus role confusion (Côté & Levine, 2014, Gregg, 2007, Wong, Hall, Justice, & Hernandez, 2015) and is therefore a critical time in the process of identity formation, even though the process is a life-long quest (Kroger, Martinussen, & Marcia, 2010, Ryan & Deci, 2012). Before delving into the family system, it is important to situate adolescent development within the broader ecosystemic reality using Bronfenbrenner's (1986) ecological model (Wong et al., 2015). As individuals, we evolve within a number of concentric systems from proximal to distal that are key to the development of our identity. The microsystem includes our family and our peer group, the exosystem includes extended family and the community, and the macrosystem includes cultural values and customs. All these systems interact with each other. For the purpose of this article, we focus on the family system to highlight its importance in identity formation and meaning making, notwithstanding the important contributions of all the other systems.

While trying to define the notion of *identity*, Lawler (2015) stated that it hinges on the combination of sameness and difference. One of the core concepts of Bowen (1985) family systems theory is the concept of differentiation of self or individuation. It refers to the ability of family members to express their own individuality and act autonomously while remaining emotionally connected to others. It also refers to the degree to which difference is tolerated with the family system (Anderson & Sabatelli, 2011). Before elaborating further on these construct, it is primordial to acknowledge the ethnocentric biases in the family therapy literature (Guzder, 2011). First of all, the concept of family in itself can be viewed differently in more Eastern collectivist cultures compared to more Western individualist cultures. Moreover, the concept of discovering and celebrating one's unique self and being that self without anxiety in relationship with others can reflect value-laden cultural biases (Ryan & Deci, 2012).

However, differentiation of self, which is a dynamic process throughout the life span, travels along a continuum between a need for a certain level of autonomy and a need for connection and a sense of belonging (Anderson & Sabatelli, 2011). With great care not to use the spectrum as a pathologizing tool for individual and families, the concept of differentiation of self can be a useful tool to frame our understanding of identity formation of the individual within the family system. Because identity is a multifaceted and constantly evolving construct, many elements and influences add layers to the complexity of the identity formation process. Some of the main influences we would like to explore further are the process of migration and the development of a bicultural identity as well as the impact of losses and traumas from having been exposed to war-related violence.

Cultural identity formation

The process of migration renders the constructs of culture and cultural identity formation more salient. As is the concept of identity, cultural identity is a transitional phenomenon that is constantly evolving through endless mechanisms of individuation (Guzder, 2011). Migration requires hybrid identification between bicultural worlds for all family members (Guzder, 2011). In situations in which community and family protection has been undermined, adolescents are particularly at risk during their quest toward identity and finding a sense of belonging (Hassan et al., 2015). Hassan et al. (2015) describe the construct of shifting identities and loyalties in displaced persons and its impact on their social networks and relationships. A number of factors will affect the speed of assimilation and acculturation processes, including age. Different speed of acculturation within family members will create tensions and a need to adapt and shift identity not only at the individual level but also at family system level. Research shows that bicultural identity is particularly challenging in adolescence as they might be too young to completely identify with their country of origin and too old to identify completely with the culture of the host country. This process is associated with intergenerational strains (Sleijpen, Boeije, Kleber, & Mooren, 2016).

The concept of third individuation (Akhtar, 1995) has been described to frame the possibilities of adolescence immigration—positioning oneself somewhere between the identity of the country of origin and the country of migration. Similar to the differentiation of self within the family, Akhtar (1995) describes the need for closeness and distance between the bicultural polarities as leading to a quest for optimal balance between the two "mother" cultures. Coupled with the disruptions to cultural, familial, educational, and occupational connections, refugees face numerous threats to their identity and self-concept. Refugee youth often experience a disrupted sense of self or identity that may be further affected for those who lack close sustained relationships and experience cultural identity conflict (i.e., between the values of their country of origin and host country).

Significant losses and meaning making

How do adolescents and their families grieve and make meaning of losses? How are their expressions of distress linked to these multiple, complex losses? Overall consideration of the challenges and losses experienced by adolescents affected by conflict and their families provides an important broader context for understanding and supporting their expressions of distress.

War-affected youth and families experience numerous losses (Hassan, 2015; Jones, 1998, 2008, 2014; Measham et al., 2014). These include external individual losses such as home, family members, friends; and other collective losses such as community, language, culture, and country. Refugees also report internal losses such as control, autonomy, security, identity, sense of belonging, and meaning of life (Jones, 2014). War displacement and camps further compound the effects of these losses. Moreover, collective losses may affect the space for adolescents to express their individual grief (Jones, 1998). Eisenbruch (1988) emphasizes the need to carry out grief work with war-affected youth postmigration and to be wary of encouraging rapid acculturation. He relates that interventions should allow youth to consolidate their own cultural identity and retrieve a little of what they have lost to prevent uncompleted grieving and allow for cultural bereavement.

Adolescents may also experience the psychological absence of parents who are very overwhelmed themselves by the magnitude of their losses. In a report called *Invisible Wounds* (Save the Children, 2017), 85% of adults stated "poor parenting" is a significant and rising problem. Family members reported that they did not feel prepared to support children facing such exposure to trauma due to the conflict. Parents reported that they felt helpless, and many parents stated they lacked the time and ability to support their children and help them deal with distress (Save the Children, 2017).

On the other hand, Syrian adolescents in Jordan reported that talking to parents and friends was their most common coping mechanism (International Medical Corps & UNICEF, 2013). The family can provide ways of coping and buffer the potential negative emotional consequences of violence exposure during war and displacement (Hassan et al., 2015). As mentioned above, this buffering is mitigated by the caretakers struggling themselves with emotional distress, and the adolescents not always disclosing their own struggle by fear of overburdening their already overwhelmed parents (Hassan et al., 2015, International Medical Corps & UNICEF, 2013).

Understanding the multiple losses experienced by individuals and families is primordial in putting into context the symptoms that might be reported. Mental health professionals should be careful not to over-diagnose mental disorders among displaced adolescents without taking into account the broader narrative surrounding their circumstances (Hassan et al., 2015). Moreover, clinicians should be aware that screening tools tend to focus on symptoms of pathology, with little attention to local cultural idioms of distress and to resilience and coping (Hassan et al., 2015). As described prior, individuals employ narratives to develop and sustain a sense of personal unity and purpose and coherence of identity (Singer, 2004). De Haene, Rousseau, Kevers, Deruddere, and Rober (2018) emphasize trauma narration as the reconstruction of continuity and meaning at the family level. The narration process involves multilayered meaning systems and interactive dynamics between family members (De Haene et al., 2018). Illustrations of challenges experienced by youth and their families underline the importance of systemic and cultural work in unpacking complex and dynamic interactions between the adolescent, the family and culture. Constructs of postmigration cultural identity formation in youth and losses are explored through case studies from a cultural consultation service.

Case studies

Attempting to assess the psychosocial status of refugee families requires a deep understanding of events leading to displacement and the complexities related to what has been left behind. The case study approach can be a useful tool as it contains the story of a particular family's life from a personal perspective, while illustrating the rapid changes that refugees undergo including important contextual information (Omidian & Ahearn, 2000). Indeed, the psychological distress of refugees is inextricably bound with the sociopolitical context in which refugees find themselves. Thus, to gain a thorough understanding of the phenomenon, it is important to analyze it within the context with which it is situated and explore how participants themselves make sense and give meaning to their mental health. Case studies provide strong evidence for addressing issues that require deep description and "understanding of health illnesses and health care in context" (Green & Thorogood, 2014, p. 48). Moreover, the detailed qualitative accounts often produced in case studies help to explain the complexities of real-life situations, providing a holistic in-depth understanding of phenomena that may not be captured through other methods (Yin, 1984). The case study approach allows critical events, interventions, policy developments, and programme-based service reforms to be studied in a real-life context (Crowe et al., 2011). However, a key drawback of the case study is that it is of course not generalizable to the broader population at large.

Cases were identified from the Cultural Consultation Service (CCS) at the Jewish General Hospital. The CCS is a Montreal-based clinical center, located at the Jewish General Hospital and affiliated with the Division of Social and Transcultural Psychiatry at McGill University. The CCS provides comprehensive evaluations and assessments of patients from diverse cultural backgrounds, including immigrants and refugees referred from primary care and other health or mental health practitioners. In cultural consultation with war-affected children and families, social workers or practitioners working with an individual or family will often make a request for consultation if they believe that issues of culture are inherent to the case, and workers require guidance to providing culturally appropriate and supportive care, assessment and treatment (Guzder, 2014, Measham et al., 2014).

Ethical approval was received from the Institutional Ethics Review Board of the Jewish Genral Hospital (Centre intégré universitaire de santé et de services sociaux du Centre-Ouest-de-l'île-de-Montréal – Hôpital général juif – Bureau de l'examen de la recherche). Care was taken to ensure the anonymity of the family and the practitioners involved by allocating appropriate codes and withholding names and identifying descriptors.

The research team initially identified 12 cases of war-affected children and families who encountered the mental health system and were referred to the CCS. Recurring themes were then identified through an inductive iterative analysis process. Through inductive analysis, researchers gain insights into patterns that exist in the social world under study that are grounded in the experiences of individuals acting in it (Glaser & Strauss, 1967). To select two instrumental case studies, the research team analyzed the interactions of themes within each case and across the whole data set to compare cases (horizontal analysis). The analysis process began by collating all the sources of data pertaining to the cases, including reports from interviews and home visits with the family as well as psychiatric evaluations. A coding scheme was then developed using this inductive process.

Through the analysis, the two main themes that emerged were (1) identity formation and differentiation of self and (2) nonspecific physical symptoms and cultural idioms of distress.

Differentiation of self

We present two stories to illustrate two possible trajectories in the differentiation of self. Names have been changed for anonymity. The first trajectory, illustrated by the story of Saya, can be described as identity diffusion or a sense of freezing in time of the identity with significant implications for the mental health of the adolescent. The second trajectory, illustrated by the story of Rasha, focused around the issue of seeking autonomy and individuation with important implications regarding tension within the family system around the acculturation process. Both stories involve 16-year-old girls, both the eldest of four children, who, despite similar family structure, experienced very different paths. For reason of space, we do not elaborate on the question of gender in the following analysis but would like to acknowledge its importance in identity formation and meaning making for these two young women.

The story of Saya

A 16-year-old Sunni girl of Syrian origin, Saya had received refugee status in Canada and had been there for a few months. She is the eldest of four children and was separated from rest of her family members who are now applying for refugee status. She has witnessed and fled from the violence and feared for her safety and her family's as they have received threats for the regime. She lives with extended family members, desperate for her family to join her as soon as possible. She is anxious about her family's precarity. As her hopelessness about their situation grew, she became increasingly unable to function, demonstrated by recent absences in school. She cries most of the time, and her thoughts are permeated by pessimistic and anxious ruminations about never seeing her family again. She is unable to focus on her classes, has ceased all leisure activities, and sleeps a lot. She describes sleep as the only way to escape her current anguish. She reports having terrifying nightmares about being sent back to Syria. Her parents are the main source of emotional support for her through daily communication. She continues to pray and reports religion as an important source of support. Her academic, social, and personal developments seem to have come to a standstill, whereas she was a striving student before the separation. The recommendations from CCS consultation were (1) family reunification in as much as possible and (2) pursuing individual therapeutic support with a social worker using a systemic lens.

The significant losses experienced by the youth, paired with the absence of her family unit, seem to have stunted her ability to proceed with her identity formation. This disruption in her developmental timeline and her family life cycle seem to negatively affect her mental health and her ability to function. Unaccompanied refugee youth are most at risk for mental health challenges (Bean, Derluyn, Eurelings-Bontekoe, Broekaert, & Spinhoven, 2007; Derluyn, Mels, & Broekaert, 2009). Derluyn et al. (2009) reported that unaccompanied adolescents are especially likely to be exposed to premigration trauma and to show more depressive symptoms upon resettlement. Unaccompanied minors show higher levels of PTSD symptoms than accompanied minors and minors from nonrefugee populations (Huemer et al., 2009), as well as higher levels of anxiety (Derluyn & Broekaert, 2007). Other mental health issues that are common among refugee youth but may be manifested in unique ways are depression, low self-esteem, stress, anxiety, and conduct disorders (Guruge & Butt, 2015). Sujoldzic' Peternel, Kulenovic, and Terzic (2006) found that parental worries about financial problems, a common occurrence upon resettlement, can have an adverse effect on children's mental health. Although Saya reflects many of the mental health difficulties reported in the literature for unaccompanied minors, including depression and anxiety, using an individual lens and focusing only on treating the mental health symptoms will only offer a narrow vision of her lived experience. Putting her symptoms and expressions of distress in context and listening to her narrative and her meaning making of her story and her family story will open a number of meaningful avenues for intervention, as exemplified by the recommendations of the CCS. Moreover, using the construct of her inability to continue her differentiation of self in the absence of the family system offers a frame of reference to understand her symptoms and functioning. As expressed by the clinician she was "thrust in a new culture without secure attachments."

The story of Rasha

Rasha is a 16-year-old girl who is originally from Iraq with a long story of war and migration. Her mother is Shitte and her father is Sunni. The family fled Iraq because of Shitte persecution to go to Syria. They then came to Canada as refugees a few years later. She is the eldest of four children. The family was referred in part because of tensions between the adolescent and her parents. Rasha reports a lot of conflict with her father who takes her phone and does not allow her to go out. In her three wishes, her first one was that her father give her more freedom. She feels that her parents to not take her age into consideration. Rasha has been exposed to extreme violence including murders and explosions. She reports that though she feels better overall, her anxiety and flashbacks seems to be activated postfamily conflict. Although she closes herself off in her room at times, she feels really good at school. She defines herself as "unique" as in little similarities with the rest of her family. Her mother reports being the only religious person in the family and asked Rasha to wear the Hijab to be more respected by boys. She wears the hijab depending on who she is with and identifies herself differently depending on the context, "If I am with an Egyptian, I would say that I am an Egyptian in order to conceal."

Evolving within her family system, Rasha is able to move forward with her process of differentiation of self and experimenting with autonomy. Even though the process creates tensions within the family system, overall, she exhibits lower levels of distress compared to Saya, despite the fact that she was exposed to many more severe violent events. Working with the family will be important in supporting the adolescent and the family through this life-cycle transition while acknowledging their journey of loss, resilience, and adaptation.

The story of Saya illustrated strong feelings of hopelessness and lack of a sense of agency. Even though both adolescents experienced loss and trauma through witnessing war-related violence, Rasha had more opportunities to assert her autonomy and to differentiate herself from her family of origin that seemed to be a protective factor. In adolescence, agency and autonomy are crucial concepts for the differentiation of self and individuation process. Research has shown that having a sense of personal control for adolescent refugees is an important resilience factor (Sleijpen et al., 2016). In a report by United Nations Children's Fund (UNICEF; 2015) on children and youth growing up in conflict, it was stated that:

> Helping adolescents and youth adapt and exercise their agency is a major focus of the MHPSS response for this population group. It strengthens their resilience and can help them develop a greater repertoire of choices in their lives. As they develop capacities to reflect on their experiences and build new problem-solving skills and means of expression, adolescents and youth have the potential to become positive agents for change in their communities. (p. 16)

Cultural idioms of distress

The second theme that emerged through analyzing the cases was the theme of unexplained somatic symptoms reporting, which is consistent with the literature stating that refugees youth may present with nonspecific physical symptoms of distress (Measham et al., 2014). One of the adolescents above reported medically unexplained urinary incompetence for a few years posttrauma, and the other unexplained headaches.

People describe symptoms and distress to others in their community in ways that enable communal understanding and acceptance through shared meaning (Im, Ferguson, & Hunter, 2017). Cultural idioms of distress are cultural responses to various psychosocial problems or distress. It indicates to others in the individual's social world that something is amiss (Zayas & Gulbas, 2012). Explanatory models refer to the way that people explain and make sense of their symptoms or illness (Hassan et al., 2015). Cultural idioms of distress and explanatory models of illness are important constructs in understanding the meaning making of adolescents and families. It offers a window into how the experiential nature of distress is interpreted through the lens of culture. As expressed by Rabaia et al. (2014):

In mental health, what is understood in some cultures has no meaning in others. This is not an issue of finding the right word in translation, or semantics, it is about a way of being, of living, of reacting to stress and trauma linked to a mindset where meaning, culture and context are the essence. (p.179)

Understanding the role that the body plays in experiencing and communicating symptoms of distress within a given cultural context is crucial for physicians and others assisting refugees (Coker, 2004). While treating South Sudanese refugees in Cairo, doctors noticed many physical complaints in the absence of organic dysfunction, often termed "somatization." During interviews, they found that pain was woven into narratives reflecting how people make sense of their sufferings, their identity, and their world. Indirect expressions of distress are common in many cultures, often expressing physical complaints before addressing psychological dimensions. In certain cultures, the physical and psychological are more explicitly interconnected in the explanatory model of illness (Hassan et al., 2015). Coker (2004) states that:

> When the self is broken apart, it hurts, and pain is the ultimate embodied metaphor.... It is found in the heart, the stomach, the head, the legs, but particularly, in these narratives, in the self, or *nafs* in Arabic (a term which refers loosely to one's self or psyche). The self, identity, and body are truly one, and "pain" was expressed by the participating informants at all of these levels literally simultaneously. (p. 17)

Clinical implications

In exploring the question—how to best help adolescent refugees and their families?—we set out to demonstrate the importance of contextualizing expressions of distress in adolescents who had to flee from war-affected areas using a family and a cultural lens. Case studies were used to illustrate the constructs of postmigration identity formation and differentiation of self describing two trajectories. In one case study, the adolescent was not able to differentiate from her family system because of their absence and the negative impact on her mental health. In the other study, the adolescent was attempt differentiation of self, causing tensions within the family system. Finally, the case analysis also emphasized the clinical relevance of exploring meaning making and cultural idioms of distress in the face of trauma and loss at the individual and the family level.

In terms of clinical implication, using a family lens will bring into focus the importance of strengthening and improving interactions within the family system whether one is intervening with individual or the family. Adding a cultural lens to the systemic lens will help better understand cultural idioms of distress as a systemic phenomenon. Each member of the family and the system as a whole, are engaged in acculturation processes, though the impact on identity and cultural identity adds additional burdens to the developmental tasks of adolescence. Because symptoms and distress may be embedded with familial dynamics and cultural idioms of distress, the aim of a therapist is to foster conditions of safety in therapeutic spaces to explore the narrative of the families and youth, as well as their meaning making and explanatory models of distress.

The goal of family intervention posttrauma is to strengthen capacity and to restore meaning and connectedness within family relationships (McGoldrick & Hardy, 2008). Panter-Brick et al. (2017) report an important gap in the literature on family and community resilience. In a study in which they developed a culturally relevant measure of resilience, 11- to 18-year-old Syrian refugees reported drawing strength from positive relationships in their community and that family relations were paramount. Following the implementation of a group intervention for adolescent Syrian refugees, Panter-Brick et al. concluded that "To achieve long-term benefits, however, interventions will need to enhance familial and structural support, as well as the individual and interpersonal support provided in current programming". (p. 538)

In a qualitative study conducted in Gaza, Liberia, and Sri Lanka with adolescents girls postconflicts, Samuels, Jones, and Abu Hamad (2017) found that supportive and caring relationships with family played a pivotal role in the psychosocial well-being of the adolescents. Al-Sabah et al. (2015) reported that a number of caregivers in Bosnia reported that their own fears and anxiety often interfered with their interactions with their children. Despite these disruptions in their relationships, more than one third of adolescents reported growing closer to their caregivers as a result of the war (Al Sabah et al., 2015).

De Haene et al. (2018) reported that an increasing interest in systemic approaches to refugee care, moving beyond the individual level and emphasizing dynamics within family and community contexts. Zooming out with a wider systemic lens, Measham et al. (2014) illustrated the importance of collaborative care between mental health and primary care providers when working with refugee families to offer a holistic approach. The importance of training of health care providers to deliver culturally sensitive care was also highlighted. De Haene et al. (2018) proposed a shift toward sensitive engagement with refugee families' unique vocabularies of suffering and coping, using the process of trauma narration. It is important to understand cultural idioms of distress as they can be an important manifestation of mental health symptoms (Betancourt, Speelman, Onyango, & Bolton, 2009). In their recommendations on how to best care for a newly arrived Syrian refugee family, Pottie, Greenaway, Hassan, Hui, and Kirmayer (2016) suggested that practitioners stay alert to associated signs and symptoms of PTSD and depression including unexplained somatic symptoms. The process of understanding the cultural meanings of these expressions is one of inquiry and using trained translators and culture brokers (Guzder, 2011).

Mental health providers need to be aware that their own explanatory models of mental health problems may not be shared with the youth or family and that imposing them might interfere with the therapeutic relationship (Hassan et al., 2015). Mental health care providers must strive to respect and integrate diverse explanatory models to optimally engage the youth and families.

Understanding local illness models and idioms of distress will allow for better communication and alliance, allowing for the mobilisation of individual and collective strength and resilience. Psychiatric labeling can be alienating and stigmatizing (Hassan et al., 2015), especially if youth and families do not feel that their stories of losses, trauma, and injustice were taken into account to contextualize their suffering. Creating a safe space for youth and families to explore their explanatory models of illness and suffering can offer the opportunity for meaning making and a consolidation of identity coherence within a broader context of connecting and belonging.

As discussed above, agency and empowerment are key constructs for adolescent refugees. The helping profession comes with issues of power dynamics, especially if one places oneself in the expert position. Seeking partnership and collaboration are significant contributors to promoting empowerment and to reduce feelings of helplessness. It involves making people actively involved in decision making of the intervention plan (Hassan et al., 2015). Clinicians as well as institutions need to develop cultural competency to foster cultural safety. Supporting systemic and family perspectives for individual interventions with adolescents post migration is important and will need to be supported not only by the clinician but also by the institutional milieus.

Conclusion

An ecosystemic and cultural lens are primordial to better understand expressions of distress in war-affected youth postmigration. The family is a natural form of support and coping and is a protective factor allowing for growth and identity formation toward a path of resilience and adaptation. A systemic model applied to individuals as well as families seen in therapeutic consultation is highly relevant in cultural work (Guzder, 2011). The narratives developed in therapy must integrate the impact of losses on identity formation and meaning making for adolescents within the family system. Cultural idioms of distress are an important window into the psychological well-being of youth and families.

One of the most fundamental human needs, other than a sense of belonging, is to feel visible for who you are. The family hopefully can provide an environment that will allow that. This need is even more pronounced in adolescence during the quest for identity. Moreover, the need to feel visible might be even more salient and acute for populations who have felt invisible through their experiences of trauma, loss, transit, and resettlement. One objective of clinical interventions is to offer a therapeutic space in which individuals and families feel visible for who they are through their own narrative and by being empowered to be active agents in their future.

Disclosure statement

No potential conflict of interest was reported by the author.

References

Akhtar, S. (1995). A third individuation: Immigration, identity, and the psychoanalytic process. *Journal of the American Psychoanalytic Association, 43*(4), 1051–1084. doi:10.1177/000306519504300406

Al-Sabah, R., Legerski, J.-P., Layne, C. M., Isakson, B., Katalinski, R., Pasalic, H., … Pynoos, R. S. (2015). Adolescent adjustment, caregiver-adolescent relationships, and outlook towards the future in the long-term aftermath of the bosnian war. *Journal of Child & Adolescent Trauma, 8*(1), 45–60. doi:10.1007/s40653-014-0035-7

Anderson, S. A., & Sabatelli, R. M. (2011). *Family interaction: A multigenerational development perspective.* Boston, MA: Allyn & Bacon.

Bean, T., Derluyn, I., Eurelings-Bontekoe, E., Broekaert, E., & Spinhoven, P. (2007). Comparing psychological distress, traumatic stress reactions, and experiences of unaccompanied refugee minors with experiences of adolescents accompanied by parents. *The Journal of Nervous and Mental Disease, 195*(4), 288–297. doi:10.1097/01.nmd.0000243751.49499.93

Betancourt, T. (2015). The intergenerational impact of war: Longitudinal relationships between caregiver and child mental health in post-conflict Sierra Leone. *Journal of Child Psychology and Psychiatry, 56*(10), 1101–1107. doi:10.1111/jcpp.12389

Betancourt, T. S., Speelman, L., Onyango, G., & Bolton, P. (2009). A qualitative study of mental health problems among children displaced by war in northern Uganda. *Transcultural Psychiatry, 46*(2), 238–256. doi:10.1177/1363461509105815

Bowen, M. (1985). *Family therapy in clinical practice.* Jason Aronson.

Bronfenbrenner, U. (1986). Ecology of the family as a context for human development: research perspectives. *Developmental Psychology, 22*(6), 723. doi:10.1037/0012-1649.22.6.723

Coker, E. M. (2004). "Traveling pains": Embodied metaphors of suffering among Southern Sudanese refugees in Cairo. *Culture, Medicine and Psychiatry, 28*(1), 15–39.

Côté, J. E., & Levine, C. G. (2014). *Identity, formation, agency, and culture: A social psychological synthesis.* New York, NY: Psychology Press.

Crowe, S., Cresswell, K., Robertson, A., Huby, G., Avery, A., & Sheikh, A. (2011). The case study approach. *BMC Medical Research Methodology, 11*(1), 100. doi:10.1186/1471-2288-11-100

De Haene, L., Rousseau, C., Kevers, R., Deruddere, N., & Rober, P. (2018). Stories of trauma in family therapy with refugees: Supporting safe relational spaces of narration and silence. *Clinical Child Psychology and Psychiatry, 23*(2), 258–278. doi:10.1177/1359104518756717

Denov, M., Rabiau, M., & Shevell, M. (in press). Intergenerational resilience in families affected by war, displacement and migration: 'It Runs in the Family'. *Journal of Family Social Work, Special Issue.*

Derluyn, I., & Broekaert, E. (2007). Different perspectives on emotional and behavioural problems in unaccompanied refugee children and adolescents. *Ethnicity and Health, 12*(2), 141–162. doi:10.1080/13557850601002296

Derluyn, I, & Broekaert, E. (2008). *International Journal Of Law and Psychiatry, 31*(4), 319-330. doi:10.1016/j.ijlp.2008.06.006

Derluyn, I., Broekaert, E., & Schuyten, G. (2008). Emotional and behavioural problems in migrant adolescents in Belgium. *European Child & Adolescent Psychiatry, 17*(1), 54–62. doi:10.1007/s00787-007-0636-x

Derluyn, I., Mels, C., & Broekaert, E. (2009). Mental health problems in separated refugee adolescents. *Journal of Adolescent Health, 44*(3), 291–297. doi:10.1016/j.jadohealth.2008.07.016

Durà-Vilà, G., Klasen, H., Makatini, Z., Rahimi, Z., & Hodes, M. (2013). Mental health problems of young refugees: Duration of settlement, risk factors and community-based interventions. *Clinical Child Psychology and Psychiatry, 18*(4), 604–623. doi:10.1177/1359104512462549

Ehntholt, K. A., & Yule, W. (2006). Practitioner review: Assessment and treatment of refugee children and adolescents who have experienced war-related trauma. *Journal of Child Psychology and Psychiatry, 47*(12), 1197–1210. doi:10.1111/j.1469-7610.2006.01638.x

Eisenbruch, M. (1988). The mental health of refugee children and their cultural development. *International Migration Review, 22*, 282–300. doi:10.1177/019791838802200205

Erikson, E. H. (1993). *Childhood and society.* WW Norton & Company.

Evans, R., & Forte, C. L. (2013). A Global Review: UNHCR's engagement with displaced youth. Geneva: UNHCR.

Fazel, M., Reed, R. V., Panter-Brick, C., & Stein, A. (2012). Mental health of displaced and refugee children resettled in high-income countries: Risk and protective factors. *The Lancet, 379*(9812), 266–282. doi:10.1016/S0140-6736(11)60051-2

Glaser, B. G., & Strauss, A. (1967). *The discovery of ground theory.* New York, NY: Alpine.

Green, J., & Thorogood, N. (Eds.). (2014). *Qualitative methods for health research.* Los Angeles, CA: Sage.

Gregg, G. S. (2007). *Culture and identity in a Muslim society.* USA: Oxford University Press.

Guruge, S., & Butt, H. (2015). A scoping review of mental health issues and concerns among immigrant and refugee youth in Canada: Looking back, moving forward. *Canadian Journal of Public Health, 106*(2), 72–78. doi:10.17269/cjph.106.4588

Guzder, J. (2011). Second skins: Family therapy agendas of migration, identity and cultural change. *Fokus på familien, 39*(03), 160–179.

Guzder, J. (2014). Family systems in cultural consultation. In L. Kirmayer, J. Guzder, & C. Rousseau (Eds.), *Cultural consultation: Encountering the other in mental health care* (pp. 139–161). New York, NY: Springer.

Hassan, G., Kirmayer, L. J., Ventevogel, P., Mekki-Berrada, A., Quosh, C., El Chammay, R., … Song, S. (2015). *Culture, context and the mental health and psychosocial wellbeing of Syrians: A review for mental health and psychosocial support staff working with Syrians affected by armed conflict* (pp. 14–15). Geneva, Switzerland: UNHCR.

Hjern, A., Angel, B., & Jeppson, O. (1998). Political violence, family stress and mental health of refugee children in exile. *Scandinavian Journal of Social Medicine, 26*(1), 18–25.

Hodes, M., Jagdev, D., Chandra, N., & Cunniff, A. (2008). Risk and resilience for psychological distress amongst unaccompanied asylum seeking adolescents. *Journal of Child Psychology and Psychiatry, 49*(7), 723–732. doi:10.1111/j.1469-7610.2008.01912.x

Huemer, J., Karnik, N. S., Voelkl-Kernstock, S., Granditsch, E., Dervic, K., Friedrich, M. H., & Steiner, H. (2009). Mental health issues in unaccompanied refugee minors. *Child and Adolescent Psychiatry and Mental Health, 3*(1), 13. doi:10.1186/1753-2000-3-13

Im, H., Ferguson, A., & Hunter, M. (2017). Cultural translation of refugee trauma: Cultural idioms of distress among Somali refugees in displacement. *Transcultural Psychiatry, 54* (5–6), 626–652. doi:10.1177/1363461517744989

International Medical Corps & UNICEF. (2013). *Mental health/psychosocial and child protection assessment for syrian refugee adolescents in Za'atari Refugee Camp, Jordan.*

Jones, L. (1998). Adolescent groups for encamped bosnian refugees: Some problems and solutions. *Clinical Child Psychology and Psychiatry, 3*(4), 541–551. doi:10.1177/1359104598034006

Jones, L. (2008). Responding to the needs of children in crisis. *International Review of Psychiatry, 20*(3), 291–303. doi:10.1080/09540260801996081

Jones, L. (2014). Grief and loss in societies affected by conflict and disaster. In *International maternal & child health care: A practice manual for hospitals worldwide* (pp. 110–121).

Kovacev, L., & Shute, R. (2004). Acculturation and social support in relation to psychosocial adjustment of adolescent refugees resettled in Australia. *International Journal of Behavioral Development, 28*(3), 259–267. doi:10.1080/01650250344000497

Kroger, J., Martinussen, M., & Marcia, J. E. (2010). Identity status change during adolescence and young adulthood: A meta-analysis. *Journal of Adolescence, 33*(5), 683–698. doi:10.1016/j.adolescence.2009.11.002

Lawler, S. (2015). *Identity: Sociological perspectives.* Cambridge, UK: John Wiley & Sons.

LeFrançois, B. A., & Coppock, V. (2014). Psychiatrised children and their rights: Starting the conversation. *Children & Society, 28*(3), 165–171. doi:10.1111/chso.12082

McGoldrick, M., & Hardy, K. V. (Eds.). (2008). *Re-visioning family therapy: Race, culture, and gender in clinical practice.* New York: Guilford Press.

McGregor, L. S., Melvin, G. A., & Newman, L. K. (2015). Familial separations, coping styles, and PTSD symptomatology in resettled refugee youth. *The Journal of Nervous and Mental Disease, 203*(6), 431–438. doi:10.1097/NMD.0000000000000312

McGregor, L. S., Melvin, G. A., & Newman, L. K. (2016). An exploration of the adaptation and development after persecution and trauma (ADAPT) model with resettled refugee adolescents in Australia: A qualitative study. *Transcultural Psychiatry, 53*(3), 347–367. doi:10.1177/1363461516649546

Measham, T., Guzder, J., Rousseau, C., Pacione, L., Blais-McPherson, M., & Nadeau, L. (2014). Refugee children and their families: Supporting psychological well-being and positive adaptation following migration. *Current Problems in Pediatric and Adolescent Health Care, 44*(7), 208–215. doi:10.1016/j.cppeds.2014.03.005

Omidian, P. A., & Ahearn, F. L. (2000). Qualitative measures in refugee research. *Psychosocial Wellness of Refugees: Issues in Qualitative and Quantitative Research, Studies in Forced Migration, 7*, 41–66.

Panter-Brick, C., Dajani, R., Eggerman, M., Hermosilla, S., Sancilio, A., & Ager, A. (2018). Insecurity, distress and mental health: Experimental and randomized controlled trials of a psychosocial intervention for youth affected by the Syrian crisis. *Journal of Child Psychology and Psychiatry, 59*(5), 523–541.

Panter-Brick, C., Hadfield, K., Dajani, R., Eggerman, M., Ager, A., & Ungar, M. (2018). Resilience in context: A brief and culturally grounded measure for Syrian refugee and Jordanian host-community adolescents. *Child Development, 89*(5), 1803–1820.

Pottie, K., Greenaway, C., Hassan, G., Hui, C., & Kirmayer, L. J. (2016). Caring for a newly arrived Syrian refugee family. *Canadian Medical Association Journal, 188*(3), 207–211. doi:10.1503/cmaj.151422

Rabaia, Y., Saleh, M. F., & Giacaman, R. (2014). Sick or sad? Supporting Palestinian children living in conditions of chronic political violence. *Children & Society, 28*(3), 172–181. doi:10.1111/chso.12061

Rousseau, C., Drapeau, A., & Platt, R. (2004). Family environment and emotional and behavioural symptoms in adolescent Cambodian refugees: Influence of time, gender, and acculturation. *Medicine, Conflict and Survival, 20*(2), 151–165. doi:10.1080/1362369042000234735

Rousseau, C., Mekki-Berrada, A., & Moreau, S. (2001). Trauma and extended separation from family among Latin American and African refugees in Montreal. *Psychiatry: Interpersonal & Biological Processes, 64*(1), 40–59. doi:10.1521/psyc.64.1.40.18238

Ryan, R. M., & Deci, E. L. (2012). Multiple identities within a single self. In Leary, MR, Tangney, JP, Eds., *Handbook of self and identity* (pp. 225–246).

Samuels, F., Jones, N., & Abu Hamad, B. (2017). Psychosocial support for adolescent girls in post-conflict settings: Beyond a health systems approach. *Health Policy and Planning, 32* (suppl_5), v40–v51. doi:10.1093/heapol/czx127

Save the Children (2017). *Invisible wounds – The impact of six years of war on the mental health of Syria's children*. Retrieved from https://www.savethechildren.ca/wp-content/uploads/2017/03/Invisible-Wounds-FINAL-020317.pdf.

Singer, J. A. (2004). Narrative identity and meaning making across the adult lifespan: An introduction. *Journal of Personality, 72*(3), 437–460. doi:10.1111/j.0022-3506.2004.00268.x

Sleijpen, M., Boeije, H. R., Kleber, R. J., & Mooren, T. (2016). Between power and powerlessness: A meta-ethnography of sources of resilience in young refugees. *Ethnicity & Health, 21*(2), 158–180. doi:10.1080/13557858.2015.1044946

Stevens, G. W., & Walsh, S. D. (2016). Deepening our understanding of risk and resilience factors for mental health problems in refugee youth: A plea for scientific research. *Journal of Adolescent Health, 58*(5), 582–583. doi:10.1016/j.jadohealth.2016.02.011

Sujoldžić, A, Peternel, L, Kulenović, T, & Terzić, R. (2006). Social determinants of health–a comparative study ofbosnian adolescents in different cultural contexts. *Collegium Antropologicum, 30*(4), 703-711.

United Nations Children's Fund. (2015). *Growing Up in Conflict: The impact on children's mental health and psychosocial well-being*. Report on the symposium, 26–28 May 2015, New Babylon Meeting Center, The Hague, UNICEF, New York. Retrieved from http://www.unicefinemergencies.com/downloads/eresource/docs/MHPSS/Growing%20up%20in%20conflict-20160104112554.pdf

Walsh, S. D., Kolobov, T., Raiz, Y., Boniel-Nissim, M., Tesler, R., & Harel-Fisch, Y. (2018). The role of identity and psychosomatic symptoms as mediating the relationship between discrimination and risk behaviors among first and second generation immigrant adolescents. *Journal of Adolescence*, *64*, 34–47. doi:10.1016/j.adolescence.2018.01.004

Wong, D. W., Hall., K. R., Justice, C. A., & Hernandez, L. W. (2015). Theories of human development (chapter 2). In *Counselling individuals through the lifespan*. Thousand Oaks, CA: Sage Publications, Inc.

Yin, R. K. (Ed.). (1984). *Case study research: Design and methods*. Beverly Hills, CA: Sage Publications.

Zayas, L. H., & Gulbas, L. E. (2012). Are suicide attempts by young Latinas a cultural idiom of distress? *Transcultural Psychiatry*, *49*(5), 718–734. doi:10.1177/1363461512463262

The essential role of the father: fostering a father-inclusive practice approach with immigrant and refugee families

Sharon Bond

ABSTRACT

Studies have consistently found that fathers continue to be excluded from mainstream clinical social work practice when clinicians do not actively encourage their participation either because of lack of knowledge of how to engage fathers or biases against considering father involvement important. This holds especially true of immigrant and refugee fathers. With the majority of research studies focused on women and their children, a tremendous gap exists for male refugees and immigrants. Immigrant males and fathers in particular tend to be either forgotten or excluded from mainstream research. A significant gender bias exists in refugee research with less attention paid to boys, men, and fathers. This article provides an overview of the essential role of fathers in child development, the barriers that immigrant fathers face, their resilience through the immigration process, and how clinicians can establish a father-inclusive practice. A review will be presented on (1) the essential role of fathers in child development, (2) demographics of immigrant fathers, (3) the shifting of paternal roles and family structures, (4) social stressors and barriers for immigrant fathers, (5) the resilience of immigrant fathers, (6) barriers for fathers in clinical practice, (7) guidelines for father-inclusive practice, using a culturally informed socioecological family systems model.

Introduction

Over the last several decades, there has been a growth of empirical literature supporting fathers' important contribution to child and family development. Research findings have identified positive associations with father involvement and child developmental outcomes across the life cycle (Cabera, Shannon, & Tamis- LeMonda, 2007; Carlson, 2006; Chang, Halpern, & Kaufman, 2007; Cookston & Finlay, 2006; Flouri, 2006; Lamb, 2010; Martin, Ryan, & Brooks-Gunn, 2007; Pleck & Masciadrelli, 2004; Stolz, Barber, & Olsen, 2005).

The research directs our attention to the specific contribution of father involvement and how their involvement serves as a protective factor for

This paper is supported by the Fonds de recherche du Québec - Société et culture (FRQSC) Regroupements Stratégiques (2017-SE-196298)

optimal child development and family life. Multiple aspects of father involvement have been examined by developmental researchers, specifically the quantity and quality (sensitivity) of father involvement and how the interactions of these characteristics contribute to the child's attachment security (Lamb & Tamis-Lemonda, 2004; Tamis-LeMonda, 2004). A hierarchy of parental attachment relationships has been identified that distinguishes paternal from maternal attachment (Paquette, 2004). This hierarchy establishes the mother as the primary caregiver, and thus the primary attachment figure, whereas the father becomes the secondary attachment figure (Feeney & Noller, 1996). Assuming a secondary role by no means undermines the essential role that fathers play to support positive mental health outcomes for all family members. Father absence is associated with negative child outcomes, affecting school performance (Hetherington & Stanley-Hagan, 2002; Hetherington & Stanley-Hagen, 1999; Kelly, 2000) and psychosocial adjustment, such as higher rates of sadness and depression and antisocial behavior found in boys (Sarkadi, Kristiansson, Oberklaid, & Bremberg, 2008). These findings provide ample support for the importance of father involvement in children's development of attachment security during the formative childhood years.

Despite these advances in understanding the importance of father-involvement, fathers remain dramatically under-represented in the parenting and family literature and continue to not be considered as central to family life as mothers (Panter-Brick et al., 2014; Skinner, Johnson, & Snyder, 2005). This holds especially true of immigrant and refugee fathers (Este & Tachble, 2009). With the majority of research studies focused on women and their children, a tremendous gap exists for male refugees and immigrants. A recent systematic scoping review identifies 95% of research on refugee and displaced populations focused on women and girls with only 5% on refugee men and boys (Affleck, Selvadurai, & Sikora, 2018). Immigrant males and fathers in particular tend to be either forgotten or excluded from mainstream research with mothers considered the only important caregiver. A significant gender bias exists in refugee research with less attention paid to boys and men (Affleck, Selvadurai, et al., 2018). Fathers continue to be excluded from mainstream clinical social work practice when clinicians do not actively encourage their participation, either due to a lack of knowledge on how to engage fathers or biases against considering father involvement important. (Phares, Fields, & Binitie, 2006).

This article provides a selected review of the literature on immigrant fathers, their essential role in family life and the importance of their inclusion in clinical practice with families. Rather than focusing on immigrants and refugees from certain geographic areas, this article provides a broad sweep of immigrants, offering a framework to understand the immigration trajectory with its impact on family life rather than a focus on a specific geographical area. Additionally, this article provides an overview of the essential role of fathers in child development, the demographics of immigrant fathers, the shifting of paternal roles and family structures with immigration, the stressors and barriers that they face alongside their resilience, and the specific barriers in clinical practice. Finally, this article concludes by offering guidelines for a father-inclusive practice, using a culturally informed socioecological family systems model.

Father's essential role in child development

It is widely understood that fathers make a difference in the lives of their children, and active father involvement is the core ingredient to promote healthy child outcomes. Lamb, Pleck, Charnov, and Levine (1987) remain the most influential leaders in fatherhood research, having developed a conceptual model of paternal involvement that serves as the standard for clinical practice and research. Their model defines positive paternal involvement as comprised of three core domains: (1) interaction: the father engaging directly with his child (positive activity engagement), (2) accessibility: the father being physically and/or psychologically available to his child (warmth responsiveness), and (3) responsibility: the father assuming responsibility for his child's welfare and care (control). This model has been widely cited in paternal research and serves as a clinical guide for father-oriented practice. This concept has been generalized across cultural groups, including fathers who may live separate from their children. For example, "African American and African Caribbean men become fathers through diverse marital/mating systems. A majority of Caribbean men become fathers in visiting unions after which they enter into common-law relationships" (Roopnarine & Hossain, 2013, p. 231). Despite the different life-course arrangements and parenting practices, "the data indicate[s] that African Caribbean fathers engage in responsive care practices that are sensitively attuned to children's needs, with fathers across socio-economic groups showing reasonable warmth to children" (Roopnarine & Hossain, 2013, p. 237). Building on Lamb's early work (Lamb, Pleck, Charnov & Levine, 1987), attachment researchers (Grossmann, Grossmann, & Waters, 2005) have investigated whether there is a direct link between father involvement and attachment security. Their findings point toward a secure father–child attachment relationship as related to quantity and quality of fathering behavior, remaining relatively stable across early childhood, and an increase in paternal involvement over time (Grossmann et al., 2005).

Paquette and Dumont (2013) describe father's specific role in the development of attachment security. Fathers have traditionally been observed as forming attachments with their children through active play in contrast to mothers through caregiving roles (Lamb, 1975, 2010; Panades-Bias, 2008). Although mothers play a calming, containing role for the child, fathers develop what has been termed an "activation relationship" (Paquette, 2004). Father's activation relationship serves as a core structure for the development of a secure base relationship. Paquette and his colleagues (Gaumon & Paquette, 2013; Paquette & Bigras, 2010) developed the concept of the "activation relationship" that is the affective bond that allows children to open up to the outside world focusing primarily on parental stimulation of risk taking and control that distinguishes paternal from maternal attachment. The activation relationship that distinguishes paternal attachment is associated with father's ability to gradually challenge and emotionally support his child through developmental challenges (Bretherton, 1992; Grossmann et al., 2002).

Overall fathers' love appears to be as essential as mothers' for the children's psychological and developmental well-being (Lamb, 2004, 2010). The evidence supports father involvement as a crucial developmental standard supporting child cognitive, emotional, and social development, and positive physical health for children and their mothers (Gjerdinjen, Froberg, & Fontaine, 1991). Therefore, father involvement is affirmed through the quality of the coparental relationship, which supports the child's developmental trajectory. As a result, the couple relationship and the family system becomes an important context within which to promote and sustain father involvement. Socioecological theory provides a crucial framework for understanding and strengthening father involvement within his larger social and environmental context. This model considers the complex interplay between individuals, relationships, community, and societal factors.

Demographics of immigrant fathers: who are they?

Immigration in North America

The United States has been one of the top destinations for international migrants with one fifth of world's migrant living there since 2017 (Batalova & Alperin, 2018). More than 43.7 million migrants reside in the United States accounting 13.5% of the American population according to American Community Survey (ACS) (Yearbook of Immigration Statistics, 2017) data.

In 2016, 1.49 million foreign-born individuals moved to the United States, a 7 percent increase from the 1.38 million coming in 2015. India was the leading country of origin, with 175,100 arriving in 2016, followed by 160,200 from China/Hong Kong, 150,400 from Mexico, 54,700 from Cuba, and 46,600 from the Philippines. India and China surpassed Mexico in 2013 as the top origin countries for recent arrivals. Among the top countries of recent immigrants, many more Cuban born arrived in 2016 (54,700) compared to 2015 (31,500) – an increase of 74 percent. (Zong, Batalova, & Hallock, 2018, p. 1)

Immigrants make up 21.9% of Canada's population, thus approximately one in five Canadians are born outside of Canada (Statistics Canada, 2016).

Recent census data indicates that 53% were economic immigrants (along with their spouse/partner and dependents), 26% were sponsored family members, 20% were either resettled refugees or protected persons, and 1% was in the humanitarian and other category. Of those immigrants, 3,586,495 are males (Statistics Canada, 2016). The latest figures reveal that 61.8% were born in Asia (including the Middle East). No fewer than seven of the top 10 source countries of new immigrants were Asian: Philippines, India, Syria, Republic of China, Pakistan, and South Korea (Government of Canada, 2017). Around one fouorth of all immigrants admitted in the first 5 months of 2016 were refugees. For these men fleeing war-affected countries, profound experiences of loss, trauma, discrimination, and social dislocation are a few of many psychosocial stressors that accompany the immigration and resettlement process (Kirmayer et al., 2011).

Immigrant fathers in North America

In the United States, the National Responsible Fatherhood Clearinghouse (NRFC; 2008) analyzed statistics on immigrant fathers. The data indicates that immigrant fathers in the United Sates endorse more traditional, family-oriented values. This is illustrated through the NRFC (2008) data that reported 20% of immigrant fathers live with their child's mother compared to 13% of fathers born in America. More immigrant fathers live with their children than fathers born in America, with 6% of immigrant fathers are nonresident fathers compared to 11% of fathers born in the United States. However similar to their Canadian counterparts, American fathers face similar social disadvantage including unemployment, poverty, lack of higher education, to name a few. Immigrants are less likely to have a high school education than fathers born in America (NRFC, 2008). Infants whose parents are immigrant fathers reside in lower income families than infants whose fathers are born in the United States (Batalova & Alperin, 2018).

Based on analysis of census data from Statistics Canada in 2006, Ravanera and Hoffman (2012) estimated there are 1,041,100 fathers who are immigrants in Canada. Immigrant fathers represent slightly over one fourth of men living with dependent children. Immigrant men overwhelmingly endorse traditional family structures. For example, more immigrant fathers are married (91.7%) than native-born fathers (73.9%), and fewer immigrant fathers live in common-law relationships (4.7%) than native-born fathers (19.7%). Furthermore, immigrant fathers are also less likely to parent alone (3.7%) than fathers born in Canada (6.4%) (Ravanera & Hoffman, 2012). Analysis of census data from Statistics Canada in 2006 reveals that time of immigration to Canada affects socioeconomic measures, such that fathers who immigrated prior to 1991 report comparable socioeconomic indicators to those born in Canada, whereas fathers who immigrated to Canada more recently face higher risks for economic difficulties (Ravanera & Hoffman, 2012). The *Annual Report to Parliament on Immigration* (Government of Canada, 2017) stated male immigrants have higher unemployment rates compared to males who are born in Canada.

In 2016, 46,319 refugees were resettled to Canada, exceeding the high end of the planned admission range of 46,000. This statistic reflects the Government's commitment to resettle refugees from all over the world, with a specific emphasis on responding to the unfortunate plight of Syrian refugees. Syrian refugee fathers face enormous social and emotional challenges upon entry into Canada including uncertainty about immigration and refugee status, unemployment, or underemployment, loss of social status; loss of community and social supports and concern about family members left behind and possibility of reunification; difficulties in learning a new language, acculturation, and adaptation (Kirmayer et al., 2011). Immigration for these men is frequently associated with serious experiences of war-related trauma contributing to their appreciation and sensitivity for eventual family connection (Affleck, Selvadurai, et al., 2018).

Immigrant fathers: the shifting of paternal roles and family structures

Immigration is considered a complicated life transition that may include the shifting of paternal and familial roles, responsibilities, and major changes in the family structure. The complexity of the immigrant fathers' experience, from premigration to resettlement and postmigratory adjustment, initiates an extended chain of change and adaptation in all spheres of life (McGoldrick, 2008; McGoldrick, Carter, & Garcia-Preto, 2011; McGoldrick, Pearce, & Giordano, 2005). The traditional father role within the patriarchal family structure is often challenged with immigration as a father's authority is diminished when adults become highly dependent upon their children as interlocutors in the host country (Abi-Hashem, 2011; Mohdzain, 2011; Weine et al., 2008, 2004). Deng and Marlowe (2013) argued that refugee children often learn the new language and customs of the host country faster than their parents, and these developments may place them in the role of interpreters or "cultural brokers" between their parents and the host community. This shift can also lead to role reversal, potentially compromising the parental hierarchy and the respect children have for their parents and their authority. Studies of Vietnamese adolescents in the United States reveal, "most of the adolescents perceived that their fathers have not acculturated to the U.S. culture and continue to practice the traditional authoritarian parenting style, regardless of the amount of time spent in the United States" (Nguyen, 2008, p. 337).

Migration and resettlement involves multi-layered transitions and changes in roles, culture, and language, location often accompanied by economic and social adaptation, "This migratory process typically involves three major sets of transitions: 1. changes in personal ties and reconstruction of social networks; 2. the move from one socio-economic system to another and 3. the move from one cultural system to another" (Kirmayer, 2013, p. E961). These transitions can contribute to "family relationship challenges, specifically cultural conflicts between traditional values that are collectivist in nature and American cultural values of individualism" (Ho & Birman, 2010, p. 3). In addition, transitional conflict can arise when there are differential rates of adjustment among family members. Some members can move more rapidly along the transitional pathway (e.g., "rapid assimilation") whereas others struggle to maintain the traditional culture at all costs (Landau, 1982; Roer-Strier, 1996; Lamb & Bougher, 2009). Acculturation occurring within a short time period can have negative consequences when there has been a rapid shift from traditional to egalitarian values, or a distancing from the core values and belief system of their cultural heritage. The otherwise stabilizing effect of family values can become eroded in families that have fewer resources to access during the postimmigration transition period (Lamb & Bougher, 2009).

Refugee and immigrant families affected by war can present with cultural variations of authority and extended family descent patterns (sometime arriving from countries that have polygamous family structures-arranged or semiarranged marriages) challenging Western concepts of the legal Canadian family. Families of war often experience fragmentation, including the loss of the primary familial leadership with children, traditional kinship systems, caregivers and/or community members called upon to serve as replacement authority figures and parental overseers (Baker, 2014; Baker & Albanese, 2009). War-induced migration also typically involves "family separation" with physical relocation separating individuals from extended family systems, nuclear families, or at minimum community or friendship circles.

In addition to the above, these families face increased exposure to violence, susceptibility to exploitation, heightened poverty, economic insecurity, and feelings of cultural and linguistic isolation (Laban, Gernaat, Komproe, van der Tweel, & De Jong, 2005; Nickerson, Steel, Bryant, Brooks, & Silove, 2011; Rousseau, Mekki-Berrada, & Moreau, 2001). The sense of displacement and related lack of trust in social institutions can further intensify dependence on the family unit and create a need for maintaining cultural continuity. Family systems theory provides a framework for understanding how migration intersects with the life cycle process, with heightened stress at pivotal developmental life-course transitions (Nichols & Davis, 2017). Systems theory places its conceptual focus on the family system as a whole with attention to the wider social ecology. Individual behavior is understood within the context of multiple overlapping systems including the broader social context.

Social stressors and barriers for immigrant fathers

Premigration trauma

Men's experiences of premigratory trauma are often overlooked. It is important to highlight a gap in our understanding of men's premigratory trauma. Studies have underscored that some men's experiences of premigration trauma are often more extreme than for women. For example, in times of war, men are often subjected to greater (in numbers and in intensity) traumatic events such as physical combat, assault, combat, injury, and witnessing violent injury and death (Tolin & Foa, 2006). Men are also subjected to more torture and imprisonment, often for longer duration than women (Abu-Ras & Suarez, 2009). Like women, men are also subjected to sexual violence and sexual torture during war, often at shockingly high rates (Affleck, Selvadurai, et al., 2018). Premigratory trauma has a direct effect on caregiving and parenting capacity for fathers; thus male trauma and postmigratory adjustment is an important area of focus (Van Ee, Sleijpen, Kleber, & Jongmans, 2013).

Acculturation stress

Higher acculturation to North American societal norms in terms of language, citizenship, and self-identification is often associated with poorer mental health outcomes for children (e.g., depression or drug and alcohol abuse) (Alegría et al., 2008; Organista, 2007; Vega et al., 1998). As previously discussed, the different pacing of the acculturation process among refugee and immigrant parents and their children can lead to the rise of "acculturative distance." The rise of this distance can be fostered by a mismatch between parents striving to maintain and endorse their own cultural practices, in contrast to their children who tend to embrace the cultural attitudes and behaviors of the host country (Kwang & Wood, 2009; Suanet & Van de Vijver, 2009). . The increase of acculturative distance can contribute to communication problems in the family, including cut-off and difficulty reestablishing satisfactory parent–child relations (Ho, 2014; Ying & Han, 2007).

Acculturation difficulties can include heightened gender-role conflicts including issues related to ethnic and religious identity and intergenerational conflict within the family. For fathers specifically, the changes in gender roles postmigration can be particularly stressful and can include the following experiences: the lessening of responsibility and power differentials in relation to their wives, feelings of disappointment (e.g., depression and low self-esteem), limited work opportunities (e.g., exclusion from professional employment, lack of achievement), and discrimination and social exclusion (Noh, Kaspar & Wickrama, 2007). These changing family roles are often accompanied by the decline in self-esteem due to unemployment, poverty, and loss of social status. These inter-related factors have been linked with higher rates of paternal depression and acute feelings of grief, loss, guilt, isolation, and marginalization; increased alcohol intake; and a rise in disciplinary and neglectful behavior toward children (Strier & Roer-Strier, as cited in Lamb, 2010, p. 436). Ultimately, fathers who suffer from depression and or posttraumatic stress disorder are significantly compromised in their caregiving capacity, which has a direct effect on child developmental outcomes (Panter-Brick et al., 2014).

Underemployment, unemployment, role reversal, social isolation, and discrimination

Studies have found (Colic-Peisker & Tilbury, 2007; Nickerson et al., 2011) that issues of underemployment and the shame associated with the lack of social standing can be especially difficult for refugee men, as they often serve to undermine men's sense of identity and self-worth. Lack of employment, and the accompanying role reversal in the context of their wives employment status, can be particularly humiliating for the immigrant father and can be accompanied by feelings of social exclusion and dislocation. Western egalitarian societal roles for women including increased responsibility with shared decision making represents a cultural value shift that can contribute to heightened marital conflict, and elevated risk of spousal violence and separation. The stressors associated with fathers' inability to fulfill these traditional gender roles are not to be overlooked (Vitlae & Ryde, 2016). Some fathers face enduring social barriers to advancement fueled by exclusionary policies, discrimination, and racism (Noh, Kaspar, & Wickrama, 2007).

Ambiguous loss

An important and distinctive feature of the refugee and immigrant experience is unprocessed and ambiguous loss. Ambiguous loss theory was developed by Pauline Boss (1999, 2004) and refers to the psychological construct that can be applied to any family member or person who is "there but not there." Her seminal research has been applied to soldiers missing in action, families living with members suffering from Alzheimer's disease, or varied types of war-related losses.

Furthermore, war refugees have experienced a sense of "cultural bereavement" often including numerous losses physical and psychological. These can include the death of family members, destruction of their homes, loss of important careers and employment, as well as symbolic losses such as the one's sense of home and country, belonging, social cohesion, and connection. Boss (2004) posits that these significant losses leave immigrants in an "ongoing state of ambiguity and uncertainty interfering with their capacity to mourn this loss and move forward" (p. 553). Living with ambiguity and uncertainty may interfere with the family's task of processing and working through their loss. For fathers, these losses remain particularly salient. It should be argued that even when immigrant fathers were well prepared for the parenting tasks in their country of origin, their parenting capacity is potentially compromised by the different conditions and challenges of adapting to a new society (Strier & Roer-Strier, 2010).

The resilience of immigrant fathers

Although the literature has largely focused on the cumulative psychological and social stressors for these fathers, the strength of these men and their families is often by-passed in favour of a deficit-driven framework:

> Instead of the pessimistic prophecy of family disintegration, studies reflect the myriad ways in which new immigrant family patterns are shaped and strengthened by cultural meanings and social practices brought from their home countries, as well as by social, economic and cultural forces in the host country. (Strier & Roer-Strier as cited in Lamb, 2010, p. 437).

Immigrant fathers typically arrive in a new country with the goal of establishing a better life for their children and family (Suarez-Orozco & Suarez-Orozco, 2001). Some men attribute their role as fathers as a primary source of pride, providing them a sense of renewed purpose and heightened status in their social community (Shimoni, Este, & Clark, 2003). Immigration and resettlement can equally offer hope and optimism for a better life, which initially can have a positive effect on well-being (Kirmayer et al., 2011). This improved well-being may even better fathers' social and economic conditions, which in turn allow them to better perform their roles (Strier and Roer-Strier as cited in Lamb, 2010). Studies highlight immigration as positively related to family cohesion and improved outcomes for children, strengthened by close-knit family-centered communities, which offer the possibility of cultural and social continuity (Singh, McBride, & Kak, 2015; Treas & Mazumdar, 2004). Positive role models and the strength of ethnic pride and social support can counteract the stressors related to poverty, discrimination, and racism (Beiser, Dion, Gotowiec, Hyman, & Vu, 1995; Beiser, Hou, Heyman, & Tousignant, 2002; Kirmayer, 2013). These factors underscore how the immigration and resettlement process itself can provide an opportunity for individual growth and family development.

Father attachment

Narratives of paternal affiliation, love, and caring are often overlooked in favor of a pathological focus of father attachment. In an Israeli study comparing Ethiopian and former Soviet Union immigrant fathers' adjustment to Israeli society, a key theme identified was their strong belief in family and the importance of ensuring a sense of family well-being and cultural continuity over the generations (Strier & Roer-Strier, 2005). Although it is important to note that there were cultural distinctions in their understanding of paternal involvement and definitions of *fatherhood*, these fathers reported a deep sense of commitment and attachment for their families. Fathers' love and attachment for their children serve as a strong protective factor for their children's developmental well-being across the life cycle (Lamb, 2004, 2010; Lamb et al., 1987) and adaptive acculturation into the host society.

Developmental and attachment researchers highlight that though fathers do love differently from mothers, their involvement remains no less essential (Lamb, 2010; Paquette & Dumont, 2013; Pruett, 2000). This finding was supported by a qualitative Canadian study of 24 immigrant fathers across several cultural groups (i.e., Chinese, South American, Eastern European, and South East Asian) with the objective of gaining a deeper understanding of the internal emotional processes these fathers had about fatherhood (Shimoni et al., 2003). What surfaced was their deep-felt sense of emotional connection to their children and families, whom they considered a source of pride, adding meaning to their lives. These fathers viewed their paternal roles as a guide, educator, and mentor for their children as essential toward their well-being over time (Shimoni et al., 2003). The connection to strong family values, deeply embedded paternal affiliation, and belief in continuity in their paternal role was considered a consistent finding for fathers across cultural groups.

Understanding the immigrant father in context: a shift in thinking

Working with immigrant families requires a shift in thinking from Eurocentric models of understanding to collectivist assumptions regarding norms and standards of healthy family functioning (Guzder, 2015). Undiscriminating applications of Western theoretical models of immigrant and minority families can undermine or "pathologize these families minimizing their cohesiveness, resilience and strength" (Guzder, 2015, p. 146). Existing models for conceptualizing fatherhood are largely based on Eurocentric models of American middle-class samples and can unwittingly lead to erroneous conclusions or at worst destructive understandings of the refugee or immigrant experience (Ball & Daley, 2012; Cabrera & Bradley, 2012; Roopnarine, 2013).

Families can be understood along two principal developmental pathways, either individualistic or collectivistic (Falicov, 1983; Guzder, 2015). Eurocentric frameworks are primarily based on individualistic models whereas collectivist standards reflect the interdependence between the individual, family and the larger community network. Roles and obligations are tightly embedded within a matrix of wider intergenerational affiliations, with adherence to strict gender-role definitions, and family legacies linked to social class and ethnic and cultural affiliations (Guzder, 2014). These strong family values support the belief in family cohesion and role modelling for their developing children including adherence to more hierarchical family structures and organization. The honor and pride rooted in a gendered patriarchal position needs to be far better understood by Western health care providers, rather than adopting a critical judgemental stance that privileges the Euro-American standard as the exclusive referential framework.

Barriers for father inclusion in clinical practice

Despite robust evidence for the importance of fathers in child development, research on parenting has predominantly focused on mothers with fathers seen as peripheral to family. In fact, research designs refer to fathers as "alternative caregivers," further marginalizing their important role in child development (Gill, Dishion, & Shaw, 2014). Most parenting programs are based on social constructs that favor mother-based child-rearing practices. Interventions are often slanted toward a mother-oriented practice model, and family-based interventions are typically predicated on a father-deficit model. Namely, this model emphasizes that fathers are ineffective or neglectful in the arena of child and family development. This deficit model of father involvement constitutes the majority of parenting interventions in the United Kingdom and the United States (Panter-Brick et al., 2014).

Barriers to engaging men as parents work against father inclusion as well as father retention. Additionally, coparenting is undervalued when contrasted with mothering. Robust evaluations of father participation and the impact of fathers on child or family outcomes are hindered by the ways in which parenting interventions are currently designed, delivered, and evaluated (Panter-Brick et al., 2014). Many of the parenting programs are predominantly designed for women, with the needs of fathers minimally addressed (Barlow & Shimoni, 2000). Women typically staff these programs, which could further explain men's discomfort with these services in a setting designed to service women's issues, as well as perhaps a reluctance or lack of training of female therapists to address the issues of men.

Immigrant men and clinical practice

Immigrant and refugees men are less likely to access mental health and social services than North American born men. It is very common for immigrant men to be mistrustful of health care providers and fearful of being misunderstood (Affleck, Selvadurai, et al., 2018; Kirmayer, 2013). Clinicians need to be particularly mindful of gendered expression of distress and how men may camouflage their pain and suffering with the need to appear independent and strong. Failure to address men's emotional experiences of immigration, social dislocation, and resettlement unwittingly reinforces false social attitudes and beliefs surrounding men's invulnerability that contribute to the exclusion of men from clinical research and practice. Additionally, clinicians often neglect to look for sexual abuse in male immigrants and refugees or recognize trauma symptoms in men (Oosterhoff, Zwanikken, & Ketting, 2004). These symptoms are under-reported as men are less likely to report sexual trauma due to shame and stigma (Affleck, Selvadurai, et al., 2018). They contribute to men's reluctance to disclose premigratory trauma—marital and sexual violence. Trauma survivors' reluctance to disclose traumatic material from the past runs contrary to Western notions of openness and sharing as a necessaary pathway toward healing, and is well documented in the literature (Dalgaard & Montgomery, 2015). The creation of a secure client–therapist relationship that includes a modulated pacing of disclosure, is recommended when working with traumatized refugee men and their families.

Men's reluctance to access treatment can also be explained through culturally embedded notions of male masculinity (Affleck, Thamotharampillai, Jeyakumar, & Whitley, 2018). Internalized beliefs of masculine identity can contribute to the man's desire to deal with problems independently. Masculine incidents of distress are typically expressed through alcohol and substance use, financial mismanagement as well as increased anger, control and propensity for interpersonal conflict and violence. These behaviors are particularly present in traditional societies with high gender inequality, where divorce is not culturally accepted and there are limited work options for women (Pedersen, Tremblay, Errázuriz, & Gamarra, 2008).

There are several vulnerabilities of the refugee and immigration experience that are unique to men: the loss of the provider and protector role, the stigma of being dependent on social services and relief agencies, and the lack of self-determination that accompanies the immigration trajectory can separate men from their traditional masculine identities, roles, and relations. When these experiences accumulate, it can lead to feelings of inadequacy and failure and may trigger mental health issues. For example, there is a high correlation between unemployment and mental health issues for men but not for women (Johansson Blight, Ekblad, Persson, & Ekberg, 2006). A recent qualitative study exploring mental health and resilience amongst Sri Lankan Tamil refugee men in Canada identified four specific themes (Affleck, Thamotharampillai, et al., 2018, p. 1):

(i) Gendered helplessness of war: male participants commonly reported ongoing negative rumination regarding experiences where they were unable to adequately protect loved ones from physical suffering or death;

(ii) Reduced capacity: participants frequently felt unable to fulfill culturally sanctioned duties, such as supporting their family, due to ongoing pre- and post-migratory stress;
(iii) Redundancy: many participants felt that they were useless in Canada, as they could not fulfill typical masculine social roles (e.g. provider) due to factors such as unemployment and underemployment;
(iv) Intimate criticism: some participants reported that their spouses would often attempt to "shame" them into greater achievement by constantly reminding them of their failure.

For many immigrant men, the loss of one's way of life that follows immigration and resettlement is particularly acute. Unlike women's gender roles such as child rearing and cooking, men's roles are likely to be lost through relocation (Johansson Blight et al., 2006; Lamb & Bougher, 2009). Additionally, men can experience discrimination from health practitioners with services that exclusively target women's vulnerability, leaving men feeling misunderstood or unwanted by helping professionals (Lwambo, 2013). Ultimately, this can translate into structural or cultural barriers that impede men from accessing services. Additional factors such as lack of mobility or ability to take time off work and distances from treatment centers, lack of linguistically accessible services, concern that problems will not be understood by health practitioners because of cultural or linguistic differences, and fear of deportation and stigmatization contribute to poor clinical uptake by men (Shimoni et al., 2003). A more productive framework is a socioecological model that focuses on the social, economic, and political environments that shape father engagement with their children and families (Carlson & McLanahan, 2002; Cowan, Cowan, Pruett, & Pruett, 2005).

Guidelines for father-inclusive practice: a culturally informed socioecological family systems model

Ecological and acculturation frameworks are central to our understanding of fathers' role in the immigrant/refugee acculturation and postmigratory adjustment process. This remains particularly salient for immigrant and refugee families who face the multiple pre- and postmigratory stressors of resettlement, such as family separation and reunification, ambiguous loss, and systemic barriers and resettlement obstacles linked to postmigratory adjustment. As discussed above, all of these factors affect father involvement and caregiving capacity. Historical and cross-cultural perspectives underscore the differing roles for fathers across time and cultural contexts, distinguishing Western notions of fathering and father involvement from non-Western ideologies.

A fundamental ingredient for sound clinical practice with refugee and immigrant fathers and their families is a model that promotes therapeutic sensitivity and attention to cultural safety. The concept of cultural safety was developed by Indigenous Maori nurse educators in New Zealand, linking poor health outcomes of the Maori people in part to cultural inappropriateness and insensitivity of health services (Smye, Josewski, & Kendall, 2010). This concept has been endorsed by the Mental Health Commission (2012) as the gold standard approach to mental health practice with a focus on "issues of power, voice and discrimination as an essential complement to professionals' cultural competence" (Kirmayer, 2013, p. 366). The lack of felt safety in the social and health care institutions presents a significant barrier for effective social work intervention.

Guidelines for a cultural model that integrates cultural safety has been developed by Guzder and Rousseau (2013; Kirmayer, 2013). Clinical work with this population necessitates a developed use of self to embrace the inherent complexity of working with cultural families as a path toward cultural competence and the creation of cultural safety (Kirmayer, 2013). They stress that the therapist–client relationship forms the bedrock for work with war-affected families. Adopting a position of cultural humility, which includes unpacking meaning, suspending judgement, and increasing the capacity to listen and learn from one's clients is the core of cultural work. Guzder and Rousseau's (2013) years of training in cultural psychiatry has led to a model wherein clinicians dig deep inside the self to develop the capacity to understand the voice of the other and not directly ascribe standard Western psychological theories and knowledge as the central route for conceptualization and intervention. Guzder and Rousseau (2013) recommend the creation of a secure and safe space to exploring meaning systems with the application of several key strategies:

> Recognizing the histories and current contexts that structure inequality; embodying and enacting difference, mutual respect, and serious but playful engagement; and especially, an explicit emphasis on tolerance of not knowing as a bracketing of professional expertise, a realistic appraisal of limitations, and an ethical stance before the face of the other. (Kirmayer, 2013, p. 370)

Attention to coping styles and the unique needs of immigrant fathers further supports the provision of a culturally safe and sensitive therapeutic environment. Roer-Strier (1996) has identified three major coping styles adopted by immigrant parents: (1) the uni-cultural style maintains the traditional cultural role models of the successful adult from the home country, (2) the rapid assimilation style supports a fast adaptation to the host country norms. This is frequently associated with withdrawal of parental authority looking to the host country service providers and professionals (teachers, social workers, physicians) as the more competent social advisors for their children. This can be misunderstood by health care providers who may misinterpret withdrawal or transfer of parental authority to the experts as a lack of paternal concern. (3) The bicultural style encourages children to assimilate outside the home, to adopt the outer behaviors of the host culture, but conform to the cultural norms of the country of origin inside the home. It is important for health care providers to become cognizant of these differential coping styles with specific understanding of fathers' unique parenting role in this process.

Working with immigrant fathers and their families calls for a culturally informed socioecological family system model of practice. This framework demands a broad-based multidimensional approach that expands the clinician's perspective to look beyond the individual person toward the familial, collective, and multiple contexts. Examination of the ecological context, migration trajectory, acculturation, family structure and organization, and life cycle are used to heighten therapists' awareness about the family members with attention to their own professional and personal culture. Understanding the family within its larger social ecology, its historical and cultural roots, its meaning systems over the generations, historical traumas, social dislocation, collectivist identity, family maps of identity, and how this influences father's sense of connection and affiliation is essential for establishing the basis for a socioecological framework. It examines the diversity, which is where and how the family lives and how it fits into its environment, the family's migration trajectory and acculturation patterns. This includes the the heterogeneity of family form, where the family members came from, their resettlement processes, and their future aspirations. A family systems model places its emphasis on the family structure and organization, that is, the diversity of the preferred forms of cultural family organization and the values connected to those family arrangements (Becvar & Becvar, 2013; Falicov, 1995; Guzder, 2015; Nichols & Davis, 2017).

A father-inclusive practice should ensure that (1) services are aligned to always include the father in the treatment, (2) attention and sensitivity is given to structural and cultural barriers that impede fathers from participating or seeking support, (3) cultural safety and the creation of a secure therapeutic space remain at the forefront, (4) attention is given to social and psychological stressors related to the different phases of migration process that affect mental health, (5) attention is given to how fathers parent differently from mothers and the identification of their unique coping style, (6) assessment is conducted of men's history of premigratory trauma and the losses unique to men, (7) assessment includes an understanding of masculine expressions of distress where emotional vulnerability may be hidden or presented as resistance, and (8) attention is given to the strengths and resilience of the immigration and adaptation experience.

Conclusion

A father-inclusive model that is culturally informed pushes the clinician to attend to multiple voices and contexts, historical legacies and loyalties and integrates these cultural frames into a coherent narrative of the father's experience in the family. Father-focused practice guidelines support the clinician's sensitive attunement to the components of paternal attachment and attention to how immigrant fathers may present as autonomous and independent while hiding deeper feelings of shame, stigma regarding their inability to fulfill social-sanctioned gendered roles. The provision of a secure therapeutic environment allowing for a modulated disclosure of sensitive material serves as bedrock for culturally sound practice. A socioecological approach offers a framework for father inclusion, working with the whole family unit, rather than the separate parts of the system or unwittingly excluding the father from the therapeutic encounter. Sitting with all members of the family provides the clinician with a unique opportunity to unpack the multiple narratives of immigration, to listen to heroic stories of living in exile and resettlement, separations and reunifications, and gradually help family members process the hidden wounds and secret traumas. Through the provision of a culturally safe context, clients are free to unmask and share their personal experiences with the therapist. It is indeed a privilege to work with war-affected families to bear witness to their stories not only of trauma, but also of resilience. Clinicians who acknowledge the rich cultural heritage and heroic migration of families can facilitate the accessing of family strengths and resilience. Given the multicultural context with increasing high levels of immigration present in North America, there is an increasing need for clinicians to heartily embrace this important area of practice.

Disclosure statement

No potential conflict of interest was reported by the author.

References

Abi-Hashem, N. (2011). Working with Middle Eastern immigrant families. In A. Zagelbaum & J. Carlson (Eds.), *Working with immigrant Families: A practical guide for counselors* (pp. 151–180). New York, NY: Routledge Press.

Abu-Ras, W., & Suarez, Z. (2009). Muslim men and women's perception of discrimination, hate crimes, and PTSD symptoms post 9/11. *Traumatology*, *15*(3), 48–63. doi:10.1177/1534765609342281

Affleck, W., Selvadurai, A., & Sikora, L. (2018). Underrepresentation of men in gender based humanitarian and refugee trauma research: A scoping review. *Intervention*, *16*(1), 22–30. doi:10.1097/WTF.0000000000000157

Affleck, W., Thamotharampillai, U., Jeyakumar, J., & Whitley, R. (2018, July 12). "If one does not fulfil his duties, he must not be a man": Masculinity, mental health and resilience amongst Sri Lankan Tamil refugee men in Canada. *Culture Medicine and Psychiatry*, 1–22.

Alegría, M., Canino, G., Shrout, P. E., Woo, M., Duan, N., Vila, D., & Meng, X. L. (2008). Prevalence of mental illness in immigrant and non-immigrant US Latino groups. *American Journal of Psychiatry*, *165*(3), 359–369. doi:10.1176/appi.ajp.2007.07040704

Baker, M. (2014). Chapter 1. Variation in family. In M. Baker (Ed.), *Choices and constraints in family life* (3rd ed., pp. 1–25). Don Mills, Ontario: Oxford University Press.

Baker, M., & Albanese, P. (2009). *Families: Changing trends in Canada* (6th ed.). Toronto, ON: McGraw-Hill Ryerson.

Ball, J., & Daley, K. (Eds). (2012). *Father involvement in Canada: Diversity, renewal and transformation*. Vancouver, BC: UBC Press.

Barlow, C., & Shimoni, R. (2000). Parent education and attitudes towards mothers and the need for clarification. *Women in Welfare Education*, *4*, 59–72.

Batalova, J., & Alperin, E. (2018). *Immigrants in the U.S. States with the fastest-growing foreign-born populations. Migration Policy Institute: MPI.* https://www.migrationpolicy.org/article/immigrants-us-states-fastest-growing-foreign-born-populations

Becvar, D. S., & Becvar, R. J. (2013). Chapter 1.Two different worldviews. In D. S. Becvar & R. J. Becvar (Eds.), *Family therapy: A systemic integration* (8th ed., pp. 3–13). Needham Heights, MA: Allyn & Bacon.

Beiser, M., Dion, R., Gotowiec, A., Hyman, I., & Vu, N. (1995). Immigrant and refugee children. *Canada Canada Journal Psychiatry*, *40*, 67–72. doi:10.1177/070674379504000203

Beiser, M., Hou, F., Heyman, I., & Tousignant, M. (2002). Poverty, family process, and the mental health of immigrant children in Canada. *American Journal of Public Health*, *92*(2), 220–227. doi:10.2105/AJPH.92.2.220

Boss, P. (1999). Insights: Ambiguous loss: Living with frozen grief. *The Harvard Mental Health Letter/From Harvard Medical School*, *16*(5), 4–6.

Boss, P. (2004). Ambiguous loss research, theory, and practice: Reflections after 9/11. *Journal of Marriage and Family*, *66*(3), 551–566. doi:10.1111/jomf.2004.66.issue-3

Bretherton, I. (1992). The origins of attachment theory: John Bowlby and Mary Ainsworth. *Developmental Psychology*, *28*, 759–775.

Cabera, N., Shannon, J., & Tamis- LeMonda, C. (2007). Fathers' influence on their children's cognitive and emotional development: From toddlers to pre-K. *Applied Development Science*, *11*(4), 208–213. doi:10.1080/10888690701762100

Cabrera, N., & Bradley, R. (2012). Latino fathers and their children. *Child Development Perspectives*, *6*(3), 232–238. doi:10.1111/cdep.2012.6.issue-3

Carlson, M. (2006). Family structure, father involvement, and adolescent behavioral outcomes. *Journal of Marital and Family Therapy*, *86*(1), 137–154.

Carlson, M., & McLanahan, S. (2002). Father involvement, fragile families, and public policy. In C. Tamis-LeMonda & N. Cabrera (Eds.), *Handbook of father involvement: Multidisciplinary perspectives* (pp. 461–488). Mahwah, NJ: Erlbaum.

Chang, J., Halpern, C., & Kaufman, J. (2007). Maternal depressive symptoms, father's involvement, and the trajectories of child problems in a US national sample. *Archives of Pediatric & Adolescent Medicine*, *161*(7), 697–703. doi:10.1001/archpedi.161.7.697

Colic-Peisker, V., & Tilbury, F. (2007). *Refugees and employment: The effect of visible difference on discrimination*. Final Report: Centre for Social and Community Research. Perth, Western Australia: Murdoch University.

Cookston, J., & Finlay, A. (2006). Father involvement and adolescent adjustment: Longitudinal findings from add health. *Fathering: A Journal of Theory, Research and Practice about Men as Fathers*, *4*(2), 137–158. doi:10.3149/fth.0402.137

Cowan, C., Cowan, P., Pruett, M., & Pruett, K. (2005). Encouraging strong relationships between fathers and children. *Working Strategies*, *8*, 1–11.

Dalgaard, N. T., & Montgomery, E. (2015). Disclosure and silencing: A systematic review of the literature on patterns of trauma communication in refugee families. *Transcultural Psychiatry*, *52*(5), 579–593. doi:10.1177/1363461514568442

Deng, S., & Marlowe, J. (2013). Refugee resettlement and parenting in a different context. *Journal of Immigrant & Refugee Studies:*, *11*(Issue 4), 416–430. doi:10.1080/15562948.2013.793441

Este, D. C., & Tachble, A. (2009). Fatherhood in the Canadian context: Perceptions and experiences of Sudanese refugee men. *Sex Roles*, *60*(7–8), 456–466. doi:10.1007/s11199-008-9532-1

Falicov, C. (1983). *Cultural perspectives in family therapy*. Rockville, MD: Aspen.

Falicov, C. (1995). Training to think culturally: A multidimensional comparative framework. Clinical theory and practice special section: Cultural issues in treatment and training. *Family Process*, *34*, 373–388.

Feeney, J., & Noller, P. (1996). *Adult attachment*. Thousand Oaks, California: Sage.

Flouri, E. (2006). Non-resident fathers' relationships with their secondary school age children: Determinants and children's mental health outcomes. *Journal of Adolescence*, *29*(4), 525–538. doi:10.1016/j.adolescence.2005.08.004

Gaumon, S., & Paquette, D. (2013). The father–child activation relationship and internalising disorders at preschool age. *Journal Early Child Development and Care: Unique Contributions of Mothering and Fathering to Children's Development*, *183*(3–4), 447–463. doi:10.1080/03004430.2012.711593

Gill, A., Dishion, T., & Shaw, D. (2014). Chapter 18. The family check-up: A tailored approach to intervention with high-risk families. In S. Landry & C. Cooper (Eds.), *Well-being in children and families: Wellbeing: A complete reference guide* (Vol. I, pp. 385–406). Malden, MA: John Wiley & Sons, Ltd.

Gjerdinjen, D., Froberg, D., & Fontaine, P. (1991). The effects of social support on women's health during pregnancy, labour and delivery, and the postpartum period. *Family Medicine:*, *23*(5), 370–375.

Government of Canada. (2017). *Annual report to Parliament on immigration*. https://www.canada.ca/en/immigration-refugees-citizenship/corporate/publications-manuals/annual-report-parliament-immigration-2017.html

Grossmann, K., Grossmann, K. E., Fremmer-Bombik, E., Kindler, H., Schuerer-Englisch, H., & Zimmerman, P. (2002). The uniqueness of the child-father attachment relationship: Fathers' sensitive and challenging play as a pivotal variable in a 16-year longitudinal study. *Social Development*, *11*, 307–331. doi:10.1111/1467-9507.00202

Grossmann, K. E., Grossmann, K., & Waters, E. (Eds.). (2005). *Attachment from infancy to adulthood: The major longitudinal studies*. New York, London: Guilford.

Guzder, J. (2014). Family systems in cultural consultation. In L. Kirmayer, J. Guzder, & C. Rousseau (Eds.), *Cultural consultation: Encountering the other in mental health* (pp. 139–164). New York, NY: Springer.

Guzder, J., & Rousseau, C. (2013). A diversity of voices: The McGill "Working with Culture" seminars. *Culture, Medicine and Psychiatry*, *37*, 347–364. doi:10.1007/s11013-013-9316-0

Hetherington, E. M., & Stanley-Hagan, M. (2002). Parenting in divorced and remarried families. In M. H. Bornstein (Ed.), *Handbook of parenting: Being and becoming a parent* (pp. 287–315). Mahwah, NJ, US: Lawrence Erlbaum Associates Publishers.

Hetherington, E. M., & Stanley-Hagen, M. (1999). The adjustment of children with divorced parents: A risk and resiliency perspective. *Journal of Child Psychology and Psychiatry*, *40*(1), 129–140.

Ho, G. (2014). Acculturation and its implications on parenting for Chinese immigrants: A systematic review. *Journal of Transcultural Nursing, 25*(2), 145–158. doi:10.1177/1043659613515720

Ho, J., & Birman, D. (2010). Acculturation gaps in vietnamese immigrant families: Impact on family relationships. *International Journal Intercult Related, 34*(1), 22–23. doi:10.1016/j.ijintrel.2009.10.002

Johansson Blight, K., Ekblad, S., Persson, J.-O., & Ekberg, J. (2006). Mental health, employment and gender: Cross-sectional evidence in a sample of refugees from Bosnia-Herzegovina living in two Swedish regions. *Social Science and Medicine, 62*(7), 1565–1830. doi:10.1016/j.socscimed.2005.08.035

Kelly, J. (2000). Children's adjustment in conflicted marriage and divorce: A decade of review of research. *Journal of American Academy Child and Adolescent Psychiatry, 3*(8), 963–973. doi:10.1097/00004583-200008000-00007

Kirmayer, L., Narasiah, L., Munoz, M., Rashid, M., Ryder, A., Guzder, J., ... Pottie, K. (2011). Common mental health problems in immigrants and refugees: General approach in primary care. *Canadian Collaboration for Immigrant and Refugee Health*, (CCIRH). *Cmaj, 183*(12), E959–E967. doi:10.1503/cmaj.090292

Kirmayer, L. J. (2013). Embracing uncertainty as a path to competence: Cultural safety, empathy, and alterity in clinical training. *Culture, Medicine, and Psychiatry: an International Journal of Cross-Cultural Health Research, 37*(2), 365–372. doi:10.1007/s11013-013-9314-2

Kwang, W.-C., & Wood, J. (2009). Acculturative family distancing: Links with self-reported symptomatology among Asian Americans and Latinos. *Child Psychiatry Human Development, 40*, 123–138. doi:10.1007/s10578-008-0115-8

Laban, C., Gernaat, H., Komproe, I., van der Tweel, I., & De Jong, J. (2005). Postmigration living problems and common psychiatric disorders in Iraq asylum seekers in the Netherlands. *Journal of Nervous and Mental Disorders, 193*(12), 825–832. doi:10.1097/01.nmd.0000188977.44657.1d

Lamb, M. (1975). Fathers: Forgotten contributors to human development. *Human Development, 18*, 245–266.

Lamb, M. (2004). *The role of the father in child development* (4th ed.). Hoboken, NJ: John Wiley & Sons.

Lamb, M. (2010). *The role of the father in child development* (*5th* ed.). Hoboken, NJ: John Wiley & Sons.

Lamb, M., & Bougher, L. (2009). How does immigration affect mothers' and fathers' roles in their families? Some reflections on recent literature. *Sex Roles, 60*(7), 611–614. doi:10.1007/s11199-009-9600-1

Lamb, M., Pleck, J., Charnov, E., & Levine, J. (1987). A biopsychosocial perspective on paternal care and involvement. In J. B. Lancaster, J. Altman, A. Rossi, & L. R. Sherrod (Eds.), *Parenting across the lifespan: Biopsychosocial perspectives* (pp. 11–142). New York, NY: Hawthorne.

Lamb, M., & Tamis-Lemonda, C. (2004). The role of the father: An introduction. In M. Lamb (Ed.), *The role of the father in child development* (*4th* ed., pp. 1–31). Hoboken, NJ: Wiley Press.

Landau, J. (1982). Therapy with families in cultural transition. In M. McGoldrick, J. K. Pierce, & J. Giordano (Eds.), *Ethnicity and family therapy* (pp. 552–578). New York, NY: Guilford Press.

Lwambo, D. (2013). "Before the war I was a man'. Men and masculinities in the Eastern Democratic Republic of Congo. *Gender and Development, 21*(1), 46–66. doi:10.1080/13552074.2013.769771

Martin, A., Ryan, R., & Brooks-Gunn, J. (2007). The joint influence of mother and father parenting on child cognitive outcomes at age 5. *Early Childhood Research Quarterly, 22*(4), 423–439. doi:10.1016/j.ecresq.2007.07.001

McGoldrick, M. (Ed.). (2008). *Re-visioning family therapy: Race, culture, and gender in clinical practice* (*2nd* ed.). New York, NY: Guilford Press.

McGoldrick, M., Carter, B., & Garcia-Preto, N. (2011). *The expanded family life cycle: Individual, family, and social perspectives* (*4th* ed.). Needham Heights, MA: Allyn & Bacon.

McGoldrick, M., Pearce, J. K., & Giordano, J. (Eds.). (2005). *Ethnicity and family therapy* (*3rd* ed.). New York, NY: Guilford Press.

Mental Health Commission of Canada. (2012). *Changing directions, changing lives: The mental health strategy for Canada.* Ottawa, ON: Mental Health Commission of Canada.

Mohdzain, A. Z. (2011). Working with Asian immigrants, Part I: Far East, Southeast Asia, and Pacific Islands. In A. Zagelbaum & J. Carlson (Eds.), *Working with immigrants families. A practical guide for counsellors* (pp. 121–136). New York, NY: Taylor and Francis Group.

National Responsible Fatherhood Clearinghouse (NRFC). (2008); *NRFC quick statistics immigrant fathers.* https://www.fatherhood.gov/content/nrfc-quick-statistics

Nguyen, P. (2008). Perceptions of Vietnamese fathers' acculturation levels, parenting styles, and mental health outcomes in Vietnamese American adolescent immigrants. *Social Work, 53*(4), 337–346.

Nichols, M., & Davis, S. (2017). *Family therapy: Concepts and methods* (*11th* ed.). Boston, MA: Pearson.

Nickerson, A., Steel, Z., Bryant, R., Brooks, R., & Silove, D. (2011). Change in visa status amongst mandaean refugees: Relationship to psychological symptoms and living difficulties. *Psychiatry Res;, 187(1–2)*, 267–274. doi:10.1016/j.psychres.2010.12.015

Noh, S., Kaspar, V., & Wickrama, K. (2007). Overt and subtle racial discrimination and mental health: Preliminary findings for Korean immigrants. *American Journal of Public Health, 97*, 1269–1274. doi:10.2105/AJPH.2005.085316

Oosterhoff, P., Zwanikken, P., & Ketting, E. (2004). Sexual torture of men in croatia and other conflict situations: An open secret. *Reproductive Health Matters, 12*(23), 68–77.

Organista, K. C. (2007). *Solving Latino psychosocial and health problems: Theory, practice, and populations.* Hoboken, New Jersey: John Wiley & Sons.

Panades-Bias, R. (2008). Chapter 6: The role of fathers in their children's lives. In J. Reeves (Ed.), *Inter-professional approaches to young fathers* (pp. 179–213). Keswick, Cambria: M&KUpdate Ltd.

Panter-Brick, C., Burgess, A., Eggerman, M., McAlliser, F., Pruett, K., & Leckman, J. (2014). Practitioner review: Engaging fathers –Recommendations for a game change in parenting interventions based on a systematic review of the global evidence. *Journal of Child Psychology and Psychiatry, 55*, 1187–1212. doi:10.1111/jcpp.12280

Paquette, D. (2004). Theorizing the father-child relationship: Mechanisms and developmental outcomes. *Human Development, 47*(4), 193–219. doi:10.1159/000078723

Paquette, D., & Bigras, M. (2010). The risky situation: A procedure for assessing the father–child activation relationship. *Early Child Development and Care, 180*(1–2), 33–50. doi:10.1080/03004430903414687

Paquette, D., & Dumont, C. (2013). The father-child activation relationship, sex differences, and attachment disorganization in toddlerhood. *Child Development Research, 9*, 1–9.

Pedersen, D., Tremblay, J., Errázuriz, C., & Gamarra, J. (2008). The sequelae of political violence: Assessing trauma, suffering and dislocation in the peruvian highlands. *Social Science & Medicine, 67*(2), 205–217. doi:10.1016/j.socscimed.2008.03.040

Phares, V., Fields, S., & Binitie, I. (2006). Getting fathers involved in child related therapy. *Cognitive and Behavioral Practice, 13*(1), 32–52.

Pleck, J., & Masciadrelli, B. (2004). Paternal involvement by US residential fathers: Levels, sources, and consequences. In M. Lamb (Ed.), *The role of the father in child development* (*4th* ed., pp. 222–271). New York, NY: Wiley.

Pruett, K. (2000). *Fatherneed: Why father care is as essential as mother care for your child*. New York, NY: Random House: Bertelsmann: Broadway Books.

Ravanera, Z., & Hoffman, J. (2012). Canadian fathers: Demographics and socio-economic profiles from census to national surveys. In J. Ball & K. Daley (Eds.), *Family involvement in Canada: Diversity, renewal and transformation* (pp. 26–49). Vancouver, BC: UBC Press.

Roer-Strier, D. (1996). Coping strategies of immigrant parents: Directions for family therapy. *Family Process*, *35*, 363–376.

Roopnarine, J. (2013). Fathers in the caribbean cultural communities. In D. Shwalb, B. Shwalb, & M. Lamb (Eds.), *Fathers in cultural context* (pp. 203–222). New York, NY: Routledge.

Roopnarine, J., & Hossain, J. (2013). Chapter 13: African American and African Caribbean father. In N. Cabera & C. Tamis- LeMonda (Eds.), *Handbook of father involvement: Multidisciplinary perspectives* (*2nd* ed., pp. 223–243). New York, NY: Routledge.

Rousseau, C., Mekki-Berrada, A., & Moreau, S. (2001). Trauma and extended separation from family among Latin American and African Refugees in Montreal. *Psychiatry*, *64*(1), 40–59.

Sarkadi, A., Kristiansson, R., Oberklaid, F., & Bremberg, F. (2008). Fathers' involvement and children's' developmental outcomes; a systematic review of longitudinal studies. *Acta Paediatrica*, *97*(2), 153–158. doi:10.1111/j.1651-2227.2007.00572.x

Shimoni, R., Este, D., & Clark, D. E. (2003). Paternal engagement in immigrant and refugee families. *Journal of Comparative Family Studies*, *34*, 555–568.

Singh, S., McBride, K., & Kak, V. (2015). Role of social support in examining acculturative stress and psychological distress among Asian American immigrants and three sub-groups: Results from NLAAS. *Journal of Immigrant and Minority Health*, *17*, 1597–1606. doi:10.1007/s10903-013-9932-3

Skinner, E., Johnson, S., & Snyder, T. (2005). Six dimensions of parenting: A motivational model. *Parenting: Science and Practice*, *5*(2), 175–235. doi:10.1207/s15327922par0502_3

Smye, V., Josewski, V., & Kendall, E. (2010). Cultural safety: An overview. *First Nations, Inuit and Métis Advisory Committee*, *1*, 28.

Statistics Canada. (2016). *Canadian demographics at a glance: Second edition: Catalogue; no. 91-003-X: ISSN 1916-1832*. https://www150.statcan.gc.ca/n1/pub/91-003-x/91-003-x2014001-eng.pdf

Stolz, H., Barber, B., & Olsen, J. (2005). Towards disentangling fathering and mothering: An assessment of relative importance. *Journal of Marriage and Family*, *67*(4), 1076–1092. doi:10.1111/j.1741-3737.2005.00195.x

Strier, R., & Roer-Strier, D. (2005). Fatherhood and immigration: Perceptions of israeli immigrant fathers from ethiopia and the former soviet union. *Families in Society.*, *86*(1), 124–134. doi:10.1606/1044-3894.1884

Strier, R., & Roer-Strier, D. (2010). Fatherhood in the context of immigration. In M. Lamb (Ed.), *The role of the father in child development* (*5th* ed., pp. 435–458). Huboken, New Jersey: John Wiley & Sons.

Suanet, I., & Van de Vijver, F. J. (2009). Perceived cultural distance and acculturation among exchange students in Russia. *Journal of Community & Applied Social Psychology*, *19*(3), 182–197. doi:10.1002/casp.v19:3

Suarez-Orozco, C., & Suarez-Orozco, M. (2001). *Children of immigration*. Cambridge, MA: Harvard University Press.

Tamis-LeMonda, C. (2004). Playmates and more: Fathers' role in child development. *Human Development*, *47*(4), 220–227. doi:10.1159/000078724

Tolin, D., & Foa, E. (2006). Sex differences in trauma and posttraumatic stress disorders: A quantitative review of 25 years of research. *Psychological Bulletin*, *132*, 959–992. doi:10.1037/0033-2909.132.6.959

Treas, J., & Mazumdar, S. (2004). Kinkeeping and caregiving: Contributions of older people in immigrant families. *Journal of Comparative Family Studies*, *35*(1), 105–122.

Van, E. E., . E., Sleijpan, M., Kleber, R. J., & Jongman, M. J. (2013). Father involvement in a refugee sample. *Family Process*, *52*, 723–735. doi:10.1111/famp.12045

Vega, W. A., Kolody, B., Aguilar-Gaxiola, S., Alderete, E., Catalano, R., & Caraveo-Anduaga, J. (1998). Lifetime prevalence of DSM-III-R psychiatric disorders among urban and rural Mexican Americans in California. *Archives of General Psychiatry*, *55*(9), 771–778.

Vitlae, A., & Ryde, J. (2016). Promoting male refugees' mental health after they have been granted leave to remain (refugee status). *International Journal of Mental Health Promotion*, *18*(2), 106–125. doi:10.1080/14623730.2016.1167102

Weine, S., Kulauzovic, Y., Klebic, A., Besic, S., Mujagic, A., Muzurovic, J., & Rolland, J. (2008). Evaluating a multiple-family group access intervention for refugees with PTSD. *Journal of Marital and Family Therapy*, *43*, 164–169.

Weine, S., Muzurovic, J., Kulauzovic, Y., Besic, S., Lezic, A., Mujagic, A., & Pavkovic, I. (2004). Family consequences of refugee trauma. *Family Process*, *43*, 147–160. doi:10.1111/j.1545-5300.2004.04302002.x

Yearbook of Immigration Statistics. (2017). Department of Homeland Security's Yearbook of Immigration Statistics, and the State Department's Refugee Processing Center.

Ying, Y., & Han, M. (2007). The longitudinal effect of intergenerational gap in acculturation on conflict and mental health in Southeast Asian American adolescents. *The American Journal of Orthopsychiatry*, *77*(1), 61–66. doi:10.1037/0002-9432.77.1.61

Zong, J., Batalova, J., & Hallock, J. (2018). Frequently requested statistics on immigrants and immigration in the United States. *Migration Information Source*. Retrieved from https://www.migrationpolicy.org/article/frequently-requested-statistics-immigrants-and-immigration-united-

Index

Note: *Italic* page numbers refer to figures and page numbers followed by "n" denote endnotes.